Case Studies in General Surgery

Problem-Based Surgical Education

JOHN B. HERRMANN, M.D.

Professor and Chairman
Division of Surgical Education
University of Massachusetts
Medical School
Worcester, Massachusetts

MICHAEL D. WERTHEIMER, M.D.

Associate Professor of Surgery
University of Massachusetts
Medical School
Worcester, Massachusetts

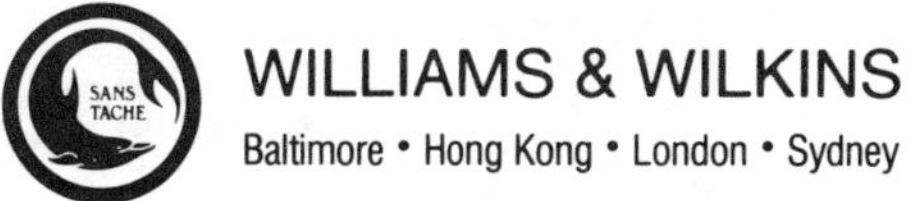

WILLIAMS & WILKINS

Baltimore • Hong Kong • London • Sydney

Editor: Kimberly Kist
Associate Editor: Victoria M. Vaughn
Copy Editor: Thomas Lehr
Design: Norman Och
Production: Anne Seitz

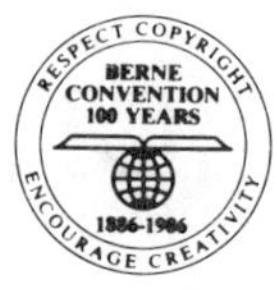

Printed in the United States of America

Library of Congress Cataloging in Publication Data

Herrmann, John B.
   Case studies in general surgery.

   Includes bibliographies and index.
   1. Surgery–Case studies. I. Wertheimer, Michael D.
II. Title. [DNLM: 1. Surgery–problems. WO 18 H568c]
RD34.H39 1988 617   88-139
ISBN 0-683-03967-9

88 89 90 91 92
1   2   3   4   5   6   7   8   9   10

PREFACE

This book is based on a case-oriented method of surgical clerkship instruction used at the University of Massachusetts Medical School during the past 10 years. This current version has been prepared as one of the components in the Comprehensive MultiMedia Program for Surgical Clerkships sponsored by the Association for Surgical Education but also has been keyed to be used with other standard surgical textbooks. The case study method as described here can be used as the basis for small-group teaching during the surgical clerkship either as an adjunct or as a replacement for the standard lecture format. The book is organized on a system-by-system basis corresponding to the chapter headings in the textbook portion of the MultiMedia Program. Illustrative cases used in the rest of the MultiMedia Program are different from those used in this volume. A problem-based alternative outline also is presented for those who wish to use a problem-oriented format. In addition, the case studies can be used as oral examination questions for medical students (or even surgical residents) and conversely can be used by students and residents to prepare for oral examinations. This volume is intended to cover the area of general surgery, including the areas of endocrine surgery, vascular surgery, gastrointestinal surgery, surgery of the breast, surgery of the abdominal wall and integument, and surgery of trauma (including burns). Emphasis is placed on diagnosis, pre- and postoperative management, and the pathophysiology and other basic science principles underlying the care of these patients. A problem-solving approach is used throughout.

ACKNOWLEDGMENTS

The authors wish to acknowledge the contributions of many present and former members of the faculty of the Department of Surgery who developed and perfected the original "Case Studies in General Surgery," many of which have been included in this volume. In particular, we wish to thank Dr. Stephen Cohn, a new member of our department, who has written the first two sections on fluids and electrolytes and nutrition which were not in the original collection. We also wish to thank the hundreds of students who have participated in this method of instruction and who have provided valuable suggestions, comments, and criticisms of both the cases and the methodology over the years. Their enthusiasm and encouragement have been major factors in publishing this book. Dr. H. Brownell Wheeler, chairman of the Department of Surgery at the University of Massachusetts Medical School, has long been a strong advocate of surgical education and has been a source of inspiration, advice, and help over the years.

We also wish to thank Dr. Peter Lawrence for his encouragement to publish these case studies as a part of the Association of Surgical Education's Comprehensive MultiMedia Program for undergraduate surgical education. Copies of our earlier case studies have been available to surgical educators through the Educational Clearing House of the Association for the past few years and have been very popular and widely distributed.

Finally, we wish to thank our secretaries, Mrs. Sue Donovan and Ms. Glenna Cloutier, who have devoted their time to typing the manuscript and, also, Mrs. Marie Ciullo, the Clerkship secretary, whose organizational work has made this project successful. We also thank the editors at Williams & Wilkins for their valuable contributions.

John B. Herrmann, M.D.

Michael D. Wertheimer, M.D.

INTRODUCTION

The case study method of surgical clerkship teaching was introduced at the University of Massachusetts Medical School in 1979 after a number of years experience with a more traditional system oriented seminar program. Although the surgical seminars were intended to be interactive, students tended to remain passive and the sessions deteriorated into mini-lectures. In addition, the largely voluntary faculty in a new medical school were widely divergent in their oganizational and lecturing skills. As a result, students lost interest and attendance dropped. Faculty responded by loss of interest in this method of teaching. Despite a better than average student body in terms of MCAT scores and grade point averages, the student's surgical knowledge was below national averages as measured by the National Board of Medical Examiners Part II Examination.

Dissatisfied with the traditional system, a case oriented seminar program was instituted in the third year surgical clerkship program in 1979. This decision was based not only on the disappointment with the traditional system, but with a favorable experience with the case method approach used for graduate surgical education (residency) and a positive impression with the method when used by other professional schools (law and business). Even during a traditional clerkship program, students tend to learn more and retain more from their contact with actual patients with real surgical problems. Unfortunately, with the compression of the curriculum during the recent past and the increase in ambulatory surgery with a corresponding decrease in hospitalization, the student has much less opportunity to become closely involved with an adequate number of surgical patients—in particular those with common surgical problems. In order to augment this dwindling supply of teaching patients, a series of approximately fifty typical case studies was developed by the faculty as a basis of the seminar program. (Later, 50 additional cases in the surgical subspecialties were added.) These case studies illustrated the critical as well as the common surgical problems likely to be encountered by a physician. A problem solving format was used throughout forcing the student to develop a plan to reach a diagnosis and/or manage a surgical problem based upon material found in standard textbooks. A series of study questions was prepared for each case to guide the student and broaden the scope of discussion. The "answers" to the questions and the "correct" diagnosis or "preferred" management plan are not given in order to stimulate discussion. The students are asked to prepare two to four cases for each daily seminar session with four to eight students and a faculty tutor or "facilitator" whose role is to stimulate and facilitate discussion, not to lecture. In this fashion, we have tried to reintroduce the "Socratic" method of teaching into the undergraduate medical eduction. The facilitator may provide certain audiovisual aids (x-rays, etc) and may summarize the points learned at the end of the session. All students are instructed to be prepared to present and discuss the case, but only one student is eventually selected for each case on a random basis. Peer pressure to be prepared is a valuable incentive. Other students are brought into the discussion as "consultants" or to present an alternative approach. Thus, a free wheeling discussion is generated with the voluntary faculty member involved in an arena where he is comfortable and knowledgeable. Role playing to reproduce real-life clinical interactions is encouraged.

The assigned case studies and faculty "facilitators" can be scheduled far in advance and can be flexible enough to allow substitutions and alternative cases in the event of emergencies. Clerkship programs with multiple clerkship sites can develop equivalent seminars at each site using clinical faculty and avoiding recurrent trips to the medical school for "lectures". During an 8-12 week clerkship with an hour seminar four days a week, a total of 60-100 cases can be discussed in this fashion covering both general surgery and the surgical subspecialties. The method encourages a problem solving approach to study and learning and is easily carried over to the actual cases the student encounters on the wards and in the clinics. Hopefully, this method will develop the appropriate investigative approach to clinical problems which will be used in subsequent postgraduate training and actual practice.

Examinations are based upon the material covered in the seminars. To base examinations on material other than material covered in the seminars would encourage students study in the more traditional fashion and not to prepare for the seminars. Despite this, a significant increase in National Board Scores was noted in our students after the Case Study Method was implemented. The case studies presented in this book can also be used as oral examination questions with the study questions used as ''prompters''. This is the technique used by the American Board of Surgery for their certifying examination (PT II). Residents may wish to use these cases as study cases for the Boards and Program Directors may wish to use the questions for ''Mock Board'' examinations to prepare their residents for the ABS certifying examination.

The Case Study Method as outlined above is not an original concept. As mentioned above, it is widely used in other graduate educational programs and has been used sporadically in undergraduate medical education for years in the form of clinical Pathological Conferences (CPCs) and other teaching exercises. During the past decade, many new medical schools have developed problem based learning curriculae to either supplement or replace traditional teaching methods. The following references are provided for further reading about this innovative approach to medical education.

INSTRUCTIONS FOR FACULTY

Implementing a problem-based case study teaching program may be difficult if a traditional lecture-seminar program has been in place for many years, particularly if the faculty (and students) are happy with the teaching program. Under these conditions, implementing a radically new program will be met with considerable resistance and probably should not be attempted without a thorough discussion among the faculty and a commitment to change. It has been our impression, however, that often among both faculty and students there is considerable dissatisfaction with the traditional passive methods of instruction, which results in absenteeism by both students and faculty. Change is welcome under these circumstances, and we have found that the case study method has therefore been enthusiastically supported by both faculty and students.

A thorough explanation of the method to the faculty is an important first step in implementing the program. The exceptional and, perhaps, the gifted lecturers should be retained in a lecture series, but most of the teaching should be accomplished through this new method. It is important not to assign former lecturers to be "facilitators" for case study sessions on the same topics that they used to lecture about. The temptation to bring their old slides and launch into the old lecture is irresistible and can only be defeated by assigning new topics and switching topics among the faculty periodically to prevent complacency. An in-depth knowledge of the subject under discussion is not a prerequisite to being a good facilitator. Being able to listen, question, guide, summarize, and stimulate are far more important attributes for optimum use of the Socratic method.

The following recommendations are provided as a guide to implementation of the case study method:

1. Obtain a consensus of the faculty that this is the method they wish to use as the major formal teaching program. Support and encouragement from the department chairman and medical school faculty are extremely important.

2. Faculty members must be instructed in the Socratic method. Many are already familiar with it, as it is commonly used in graduate education and residency training. They must be carefully instructed not to fall back to the lecture format but to encourage students to do much of the talking.

3. The course must be well organized and specific as to assignments, times, subjects, etc; but it also must be flexible to allow for emergencies and unforseen problems. There must be flexibility to reschedule sessions and to shift topics and facilitators.

4. The students must be carefully instructed as to how they are expected to prepare for the case study sessions. This should be done at the beginning of each clerkship period and reinforced periodically. Medical students have been trained to become passive learners and often arrive expecting to be taught rather than being prepared to demonstrate what they have learned. A suggested set of instructions for students is listed in the next section.

5. Faculty members should carefully study the cases they will be using. They should become familiar with the standard textbook material on the subject so that they are aware of the depth of knowledge they can expect from the students.

6. If student performance during the case discussion is to be used for grading purposes, the faculty should agree on what characteristics they will be looking for and evaluating. Depth of knowledge, reasoning, correctness of diagnosis and proposed management, and awareness of alternatives are possible areas that can be judged.

7. Final examinations—objective, essay, or oral—should be based on the material studied during the clerkship rotation. As soon as a student learns that he is not going to be examined on the material covered by the case studies, his learning will be directed elsewhere.

8. Discussion sessions should be limited to a facilitator and three to eight students, with four to six being ideal. This will allow a free discussion involving all students, without making extraordinary demands on any single individual.

9. Medical schools with multiple clerkship sites can easily adopt this method by using clinical faculty who are active surgeons at each clerkship site. Practicing surgeons (and even surgical residents) are expert at clinical problem solving, and cases such as those presented in this book are commonly encountered and familiar to all surgeons. Under these circumstances, the faculty becomes a true role model for students striving to be good physicians or surgeons.

REFERENCES

Barrows HS, Tamblyn RN: *Problem Based Learning: An Approach to Medical Education.* New York, Springer Publishing Co., 1980.

Hodgkin K, Knox JD: *Problem Centered Learning.* London, Churchill Livingstone, 1975.

Kaufman A (ed): *Implementing Problem Based Medical Education: Lessons from Successful Innovations.* New York, Springer Publishing Co., 1985.

Schmidt HG: Problem based learning: Rationale and description: *Medical Education* 17: 11–16, 1983.

INSTRUCTIONS FOR STUDENTS

The case study method has long been recognized as an effective teaching technique, not only in medicine but in many of the other professions as well. During your clerkship, you will encounter many typical and not so typical surgical cases which, if used and studied properly, will become the foundation of your clerkship experience. Unfortunately, all students cannot be exposed to a sufficiently wide range of real patients with real surgical problems in this relatively short period of time to provide a satisfactorily broad foundation in the field of surgery.

In an effort to augment your actual clinical experience, a series of case studies has been developed that covers common and critical surgical problems with which you should be familiar. These cases will be used as a basis for discussion during scheduled teaching sessions with a faculty or resident instructor. To benefit from these sessions, you should prepare each case ahead of time as if the patient were an actual case assigned to you.

The following instructions are provided to assist you in preparing the case:

1. Read the case carefully and jot down what information you will need to manage the hypothetical case and answer the study questions at the end of the case.

2. Study the appropriate material in your textbook. Use the references at the beginning of each section of cases if appropriate for your textbook, or refer to the table of contents or index if your textbook is not on the list of references. Feel free to use the library or other reference material if you wish. The faculty and residents are available if you have any specific questions about the case.

3. Write a brief analysis of the case, including the answers to the study questions. Consider various alternative ways to arrive at a diagnosis or to manage the patient. Justify your decisions. Consider alternative diagnoses and the changes in management that would occur.

4. Be prepared to present and discuss the case at the teaching conference. If you are not selected to be the primary presenter, be prepared to comment, question, and discuss the case with the group.

5. Retain your notes on the discussion along with your analysis of the case for review before the final examination, which will be based on the material covered in the case studies.

SAMPLE CASE AND DISCUSSION

CASE: **Acute Abdominal Pain**

A 22-year-old male college student is brought to the emergency room with a 5-hour history of increasingly severe abdominal pain. The onset of the pain was fairly rapid in the early hours of the morning following a fraternity party. The patient had one episode of vomiting of bilious material without relief of pain.

On examination his temperature is 38.3°C (101°F). He is pale, sweaty, and obviously acutely ill. BP: 110/70, P: 110 and regular, R:18. His abdomen is diffusely tender with nonlocalized rebound tenderness and marked guarding. Bowel sounds are absent.

STUDY QUESTIONS

1 What additional information would you like to have with respect to history and physical examination?

2 What laboratory tests would you order?

3 What initial treatment would you institute while awaiting the results of the above tests?

4 What are some of the possible diagnoses you are considering? List them in order of probability.

5 Which of these diagnoses would require operative intervention? Which would not require a surgical procedure?

6 How would you decide whether or not to operate on this young man?

7 What factors would influence the timing of the operation?

DISCUSSION

This case is a rather typical example of acute abdominal pain. Not only does this represent a common surgical problem, but it demonstrates a critical situation where the wrong decision could lead to disaster. In preparing for this case, the student should read the appropriate sections of his/her textbook covering the acute abdomen and pertinent other sections on the various disease entities that might present in this fashion.

At the time of the teaching conference one student should be selected to present the case. After the presentation, the instructor might question the student about the pathophysiology of abdominal pain, tenderness, and rebound tenderness and their significance in this case. The student should then request additional information as suggested in the first study question. The instructor can supply whatever data he wishes to lead the discussion one way or another. Other students should be asked if there is any information they would like, and this part of the discussion could be summarized emphasizing the salient features of history and physical examination pertinent to the evaluation of the acute abdomen.

The student should then be asked to list the laboratory, radiological, and other tests he would like to order (question 2). Other students might be asked to contribute, and the list might be revised to include only the studies pertinent to the case. The instructor should provide appropriate results, including a suitable x-ray study the student can interpret.

The student should then be asked to describe his initial treatment of the patient (question 3), including nasogastric drainage, administration of intravenous fluids and antibiotics (what kind? how much? how fast?), measurement of vital signs and urinary output, etc. Again, other students may be asked to contribute.

The ultimate decision—to operate or not to operate—can be discussed under questions 5 and 6. The factors in favor of surgical intervention and the factors opposed can be discussed and the relative risks and benefits examined. Nonoperative causes of acute abdominal pain should be discussed in detail, particularly those for which an unnecessary operation might lead to disaster.

The final question (question 7) relates to appropriate timing of the operation. This, of course, depends on the patient's condition, provisional diagnosis, and response to initial treatment and can be manipulated by the instructor. Construction of a variety of scenarios to which students may respond will result in an outline of the various principles of timely operative intervention.

At the conclusion of the discussion, the instructor may wish to reiterate the salient features of the case and to emphasize the portions of the case where the students had difficulty. If necessary, a further assignment can be made at this time (e.g., *Cope's Early Diagnosis of the Acute Abdomen* by W. Silen).

KEYED REFERENCES

These *Case Studies in General Surgery* have been keyed to the following basic surgical textbooks:

1. Lawrence PA (ed): *Essentials of General Surgery*. Baltimore, Williams & Wilkins, 1988.

2. Schwartz SI (ed): *Principles of Surgery,* ed 4. New York, McGraw-Hill, 1984.

3. Sabiston DC Jr (ed): *Textbook of Surgery: The Biological Basis of Modern Surgical Practice,* ed. 11. Philadelphia, WB Saunders, 1986.

4. Davis JH (ed): *Clinical Surgery.* St. Louis, CV Mosby, 1987.

5. Way LW (ed): *Current Surgical Diagnosis and Treatment,* ed 7. Los Altos, CA, Lange Medical Publications, 1985.

6. Sabiston DC Jr: *Essentials of Surgery.* Philadelphia, WB Saunders, 1987.

7. James EC, Corry RJ, Perry JF (eds): *Principles of Basic Surgical Practice.* Philadelphia, Hanley & Belfus, Inc., 1987.

Other textbooks and references may be used with the case studies by appropriate reference to the table of contents and index of each book.

CONTENTS

Fluids and Electrolytes

Stephen M. Cohn, M.D.

REFERENCES

1. *Essentials of General Surgery*—Lawrence: Chapter 6.
2. *Principles of Surgery*—Schwartz: Chapter 2.
3. *Textbook of Surgery*—Sabiston: Chapter 4.
4. *Clinical Surgery*—Davis: Chapters 9 and 32.
5. *Current Surgical Diagnosis and Treatment*—Way: Chapter 10.
6. *Essentials of Surgery*—Sabiston: Chapter 3.
7. *Principles of Basic Surgical Practice*—James et al.: Chapter 5.

Prolonged Vomiting

A 65-year-old male truck driver with a history of indigestion and heartburn presents with 3 days of vomiting. He states that neither fluids nor solids has stayed down. He has gotten progressively weaker, and now complains of dizziness when sitting up.

Physical examination is significant for a 30 mm Hg drop in systolic blood pressure when sitting up from a supine position. The patient has a dry tongue and mucous membranes, and poor skin turgor. The rest of the physical examination is unremarkable.

Laboratory studies: Sodium 148 mEq/liter (N: 136–142), potassium 2.8 mEq/liter (N: 3.5–5.3), pH 7.60, PCO_2 46 mm Hg (N: 34–45).

STUDY QUESTIONS

1 What is this patient's metabolic derangement?

2 What is the etiology of this problem?

3 Outline the steps in managing a patient with these fluid and electrolyte problems.

Polyuria

A 16-year-old boy sustains a severe head injury riding a motorcycle without a helmet. He is on a respirator in the surgical intensive care unit after a procedure to remove a hematoma from around the brain. The nurse notifies you that the patient has been urinating more than 1000 ml hourly for 4 hours.

Laboratory examination: Sodium 155 mEq/liter (N: 136–142), serum osmolality 310 mOSM/liter (N: 290–305), urine osmolarity 155 mosmol/liter (N: 300–800), pH 7.55 (N: 7.37–7.44), PCO_2 28 mm Hg (N: 34–45), HCO_3 24 mEq/liter (N: 21–20).

STUDY QUESTIONS

1 What are this patient's fluid and electrolytes abnormalities?

2 What is the etiology of this disorder?

3 Is the pH appropriate for the PCO_2? (Use the Henderson-Hasselbalch equation).

4 Outline the management plan for correction of these disorders.

Oliguria

Two days after a colon resection for perforated diverticulitis, a 70-year-old woman is noted to have a low urine output. Her serum sodium is 125 mEq/liter (N: 136–142). Her laboratory profile is otherwise normal.

STUDY QUESTIONS

1 What is the differential diagnosis of her hyponatremia?

2 What would your management be in this patient?

SUBSEQUENT COURSE

Two days later she is noted to be anuric and her pH is 7.25 (N: 7.37–7.44), PCO_2 30 mm Hg (N: 31–42), HCO_3 15 mEq/liter (N: 21–28), K^+ 5.8 mEq/liter (N: 3.5–5.3). Her blood urea nitrogen (BUN) is 85 mg/dl (N: 9–21), creatinine 5.1 mg/dl (N: 0.7–1.3).

STUDY QUESTIONS

3 What is the current acid base derangement?

4 How would you treat hyperkalemia in this patient?

Weakness and Hypercalcemia

A thin young woman is referred to your office for evaluation of weakness, nausea, vomiting, and polyuria. The physical examination is unremarkable.

Laboratory studies are remarkable for calcium 10.0 mg/dl (N: 8.5–10.5), chloride 110 mEq/liter (N: 97–110), phosphorus 2.9 mg/dl (N: 2.5–4.5), and serum albumin 2.8 gm/dl (N:3.5–5.0).

STUDY QUESTIONS

1 What is the likely diagnosis in this patient?

2 Why would an ionized calcium be helpful?

FURTHER INFORMATION

You elect to operate on the patient, and postoperatively she complains of muscle cramps and paresthesias of her fingers. Examination reveals a positive Chvostek's sign.

STUDY QUESTIONS

3 What therapy would you now institute?

4 What are the usual surgical causes of this condition?

Nutrition

Stephen M. Cohn, M.D.

REFERENCES

1. *Essentials of General Surgery*—Lawrence: Chapter 6.

2. *Principles of Surgery*—Schwartz: Chapter 2.

3. *Textbook of Surgery*—Sabiston: Chapter 7.

4. *Clinical Surgery*—Davis: Chapter 34 and 45.

5. *Current Surgical Diagnosis and Treatment*—Way: Chapter 11.

6. *Essentials of Surgery*—Sabiston: Chapter 6.

7. *Principles of Basic Surgical Practice*—James et al.: Chapter 9.

Weight Loss and Anorexia

A 65-year-old white male smoker with a history of colon cancer presents with anorexia and jaundice. He has had a 30-lb weight loss over the past year.

Physical examination reveals a thin, yellow man with bilateral temporal wasting.

STUDY QUESTIONS

1 What is your presumptive diagnosis?

2 What conditions predispose surgical patients to malnutrition?

3 List the anthropomorphic, biochemical, and immunological measurements that can be utilized to assess this patient's state of nutrition and their relative value.

Multiple Trauma and Sepsis

A 30-year-old man sustains a 50% third-degree burn as well as a severe pelvic fracture from an industrial accident. Ten days after admission he has a fever of 40°C (104°F) and positive blood cultures for *Pseudomonas aeruginosa*.

STUDY QUESTIONS

1 How much do each of the following factors affect the caloric requirement of the patient? (*a*). Fever; (*b*). Sepsis; (*c*). Severe burns; (*d*). Starvation; (*e*). Bone fracture.

FURTHER INFORMATION

The patient is placed on total parenteral nutrition (TPN).

STUDY QUESTIONS

2 Match the deficiency with its systemic manifestation.
   a. Zinc deficiency
   b. Folate deficiency
   c. Vitamin K deficiency
   d. Fatty acid deficiency

   1. Altered taste, perioral dermatitis, mental disturbance.
   2. Clotting defect, elevated prothrombin time.
   3. Scaly skin lesions on arms and legs, alopecia.
   4. Fatigue, macrocytic anemia.

Prolonged Coma

A 16-year-old boy sustains a severe head injury after a motorcycle accident. While comatose in the intensive care unit, he requires nutritional support.

STUDY QUESTIONS

1 Would you choose enteral or central vein hyperalimentation? List the advantage of each.

2 Match the complication with the modality of alimentation.
   a. TPN
   b. Enteral feedings
   c. Both

   1. Diarrhea
   2. Hyperosmolar nonketonic coma
   3. Pneumothorax
   4. Trace element deficiency

3 Discuss how medical conditions such as diabetes mellitus, renal insufficiency, heptatic failure, and chronic congestive heart failure affect your choice of alimentation.

Surgical Bleeding and Blood Replacement

John B. Herrmann, M.D.

REFERENCES

1. *Essentials of General Surgery*—Lawrence: Chapter 8.

2. *Principles of Surgery*—Schwartz: Chapter 3.

3. *Textbook of Surgery*—Sabiston: Chapter 6.

4. *Clinical Surgery*—Davis: Chapter 24.

5. *Current Surgical Diagnosis and Treatment*—Way: Chapter 5.

6. *Essentials of Surgery*—Sabiston: Chapter 5.

7. *Principles of Basic Surgical Practice*—James et al.: Chapter 11.

The Bleeder

A 26-year-old man is referred to you for a hernia repair. In addition to his symptomatic hernia, which prevents him from getting a job, he reports that he tends to bruise easily and has prolonged bleeding from minor scrapes and cuts and that he had quite a bleeding problem with a wisdom tooth extraction several years ago. He has no siblings, but he thinks he has a cousin with a bleeding problem.

STUDY QUESTIONS

1 What tests would you order to confirm or disprove the patient's statements?

2 Assuming the presence of a bleeding problem is confirmed, list the possible causes and how they are diagnosed.

3 How would each of these conditions be managed in order to repair his hernia?

Intraoperative Bleeding

You are a surgeon in a large community hospital, performing an abdominoperineal resection of the rectum for cancer on a 62-year-old insurance executive. The operation has been difficult with moderate blood loss replaced by transfusions. As the operation nears completion, you notice that all surfaces are beginning to ooze blood where a few minutes previously they had been dry. Vital signs are stable. Hematocrit is 29%.

STUDY QUESTIONS

1 What do you think is happening? What are some of the possible causes?

2 What initial treatment would you suggest to the anesthesiologist?

3 What additional studies would you order to confirm the cause of this phenomenon?

4 What definitive treatment would you suggest?

Postoperative Bleeding

The patient is a 66-year-old man who has just been admitted to the surgical intensive care unit following a 4-hour operation for a ruptured abdominal aortic aneurysm. The operation had been successful in replacing his ruptured aneurysm with a graft. Blood loss was severe but replaced with an estimated 1600 ml of autotransfused blood and 5 units of packed cells, plus about 4 liters of crystalloid solutions.

Vital signs: BP 100/60 mm Hg, P 90 bpm and regular, T 35°C (95°F). The patient is intubated and on a respirator. Initial laboratory studies show Hct 30%, PT 14 seconds, PTT 52 seconds, and platelet count of 93,000/mm. You note that he appears to be oozing from his incision and from various intravenous sites.

STUDY QUESTIONS

1 List the possible causes of his bleeding diathesis. Which do you think is the most likely?

2 What would be your initial treatment?

3 Are there any further studies you would order to confirm the correct diagnosis?

4 What would you do if the patient did not respond to your initial treatment?

Shock

Michael D. Wertheimer, M.D.

REFERENCES

1. *Essentials of General Surgery*—Lawrence: Chapter 9.

2. *Principles of Surgery*—Schwartz: Chapter 4.

3. *Textbook of Surgery*—Sabiston: Chapter 3.

4. *Clinical Surgery*—Davis: Chapters 8 and 23.

5. *Current Surgical Diagnosis and Treatment*—Way: Chapters 13, 14, and 23.

6. *Essentials of Surgery*—Sabiston: Chapter 2.

7. *Principles of Basic Surgical Practice*—James et al.: Chapter 8.

Multiple Trauma with Hypotension

The patient is a healthy and active 63-year-old truck driver who sustains massive blunt abdominal and thoracic trauma in a motor vehicle accident. Initial BP in the emergency room is 80/60 mm Hg. He is taken to surgery after resuscitation and stabilization, where the following is performed: bilateral tube thoracostomies, splenectomy, small bowel resection, repair of vena cava lacerations and exteriorization of a shattered transverse colon (colostomy). After control of all hemorrhage, transient hypotension to 60 mm Hg systolic occurs with premature ventricular contractions (PVCs) responsive to fluid and intravenous lidocaine.

The patient is transferred, still ventilated, to the surgical intensive care unit (SICU) and 6 hours after surgery becomes hypotensive again. A Swan-Ganz catheter is passed.

STUDY QUESTIONS

1 Discuss the initial management of hemorrhagic shock in the multiple-trauma patient.

2 What are the levels of automatic physiologic adjustment and compensation in human hemorrhagic shock (sympathoadrenal and baroreceptor reflexes, Starling's law of capacitance, endocrine)?

3. How do you assess postoperative hypotension?

4 Explain the hemodynamics of invasive monitoring; how do you interpret the data (Swan-Ganz catheter)?

5 Draw a chart comparing the different physiologic effects of hemorrhagic, cardiogenic, septic shock on the following parameters: blood pressure, pulse, urine output, central venous pressure (CVP), pulmonary capillary wedge (PCW) pressure, total peripheral resistance (TPR), cardiac index (CI), and blood gases.

6 How would you diagnose and treat the postoperative hypotension? What are the roles of pressors and their actions/side effects/complications?

7 Discuss the diagnosis and treatment of septic shock in the patient with multi-system failure. Discuss hemodynamic parameters, pressors, fluids, antibiotics, steroids, reoperative surgery.

Vomiting and Hypotension

The patient is a 38-year-old carpenter transferred from a local community hospital to your surgical intensive care unit because of hypotension to 70 mm Hg systolic on the basis of profuse vomiting over the previous 5 days caused by gastric outlet obstruction from his chronic duodenal ulcer.

After initial fluid resuscitation he stabilizes but fails conservative (nonoperative) management of his obstructing ulcer and undergoes antrectomy and truncal vagotomy. The duodenum was noted to be scarred and fibrosed, dissection difficult, blood loss excessive, and operating time prolonged. The patient does well initially but on the 9th postoperative day develops abdominal distension, pain, vomiting, and hypotension and is transferred back to the SICU.

STUDY QUESTIONS

1 What metabolic disturbance underlies this patient's initial hypotension? What would you predict his electrolytes and arterial blood gases to be?

2 What is the most important initial therapy (give specifics)?

3 Does this patient need invasive hemodynamic monitoring? What simple alternative forms of bedside "monitoring" are possible and appropriate? What specific parameters would you follow?

4 What is the differential diagnosis of his problem on the 9th postoperative day? Does he now need invasive hemodynamic monitoring? If so, what would you predict his CVP, CI, and TPR to be?

5 What are the fundamental principles in the management of the resuscitation and definitive treatment of a complication such as that occurring to this patient on the 9th postoperative day?

Postoperative Shock

A 67-year-old obese female diabetic with known coronary artery disease undergoes urgent cholecystectomy for acute calculus cholecystitis. During induction of anesthesia there was transient hypotension to 60 mm Hg systolic, which responded promptly to the administration of fluids. The operation was "difficult" due to inflammation and blood loss, recorded in the operative note as 1400 ml. You are the intern on call that night and are called at 9:00 PM because the patient has become suddenly hypotensive to 50 mm Hg systolic. she is alert, oriented, and has no other complaints.

STUDY QUESTIONS

1 What are the five most common causes of postoperative hypotension that could explain this patient's change in status?

2 What would be the proposed pathophysiology for this patient's shock based on each of the following five etiologies: (*a*). Cardiogenic shock; (*b*). Hemodynamic shock; (*c*). Respiratory failure; (*d*). Septic shock; (*e*). Diabetic coma.

3 What physical findings and simple maneuvers and procedures *at the bedside* would yield a working diagnosis and initial therapeutic plan within five minutes?

4 Does this patient need transfer to the SICU? Invasive hemodynamic monitoring? Reoperation?

5 Describe, in detail, the workup and definitive treatment of each of the five etiologies of postoperative shock listed in question 2.

Posttraumatic Shock

While bicycle riding, a 13-year-old boy is struck by a fast-moving automobile and thrown 50 feet. He is brought by ambulance to the trauma center stabilized on a backboard with one intravenous running, comatose, and in profound shock. There is a bleeding laceration of the frontal scalp, abrasions and contusions over the lower chest and abdomen, and an obvious compound fracture of the left femur.

STUDY QUESTIONS

1 What is the cause of the hypotension?

2 The hypotension improves only slightly with volume resuscitation and endotracheal intubation. Can neurogenic shock explain the recalcitrant hypotension?

3 What are the priorities in workup and treatment of this multiply injured boy? What sites of suspected or apparent injury, in order of importance, require urgent and specific attention to treat the shock?

4 What is your specific course of action in this patient? Enumerate your sequential actions with the expected response of the patient to each action.

Fever, Chills, and Hypotension

A 65-year-old woman with known cholelithiasis, previously asymptomatic, is admitted to the hospital with fever, chills, and jaundice, You are called to see her because the admitting nurse found her blood pressure to be 80/0 mm Hg with a thready pulse at a rate of 130 and fever of 40°C (104°F). You confirm these findings and find the patient to be confused, lethargic, and obviously severely ill. She is clinical jaundiced and her abdomen is diffusely tender with guarding in the right upper quadrant and absent bowel sounds.

STUDY QUESTIONS

1 What is your preliminary diagnosis? What is Whipple's triad?

2 What initial resuscitative measures would you institute?

3 What laboratory/radiological studies would you order?

4 Assuming that your initial diagnosis is correct and that the patient initially responds to your resuscitative efforts, what definitive treatment would you recommend?

5 What other conditions can result in this type of shock? What are the basic principles of management?

Wounds and Wound Healing

John B. Herrmann, M.D.

REFERENCES

1. *Essentials of General Surgery*—Lawrence: Chapter 10.

2. *Principles of Surgery*—Schwartz: Chapter 8.

3. *Textbook of Surgery*—Sabiston: Chapter 11.

4. *Clinical Surgery*—Davis: Chapter 16.

5. *Current Surgical Diagnosis and Treatment*—Way: Chapter 8.

6. *Essentials of Surgery*—Sabiston: Chapter 8.

7. *Principles of Basic Surgical Practice*—James et al.: Chapter 7.

Complex Wound

While hunting, a man sustains an oblique shotgun injury to his right buttock when his companion's shotgun discharges accidentally. Fortunately, no visceral, skeletal, or nerve injury is present when he arrives at your hospital. There is, however, massive soft tissue injury to the buttock with skin loss. Multiple pellets are seen in the area by x-ray examination.

STUDY QUESTIONS

1 Describe your step-by-step treatment of this complex wound.

2 How do you distinguish viable from nonviable tissue?

3 How will this large open wound be converted into a closed wound?

Wound Dehiscence

A 62-year-old woman with severe rheumatoid arthritis undergoes an emergency pyloroplasty and vagotomy for a bleeding duodenal ulcer through a paramedian upper abdominal incision. She has been on chronic steroid therapy for her arthritis. On the 8th postoperative day, shortly after the removal of her skin stitches, the wound discharges some serosanguineous fluid followed by a complete dehiscence two hours later.

STUDY QUESTIONS

1 What are some of the contributing factors in the wound healing process that may have resulted in this complication?

2 What might have been done to minimize the probability of this complication?

3 How should this complication be managed?

Suture Removal

Using your knowledge of the biology of wound healing, when would you recommend that the skin sutures be removed on each of the following patients?

1. A routine herniorrhaphy incision in a healthy 34-year-old truck driver.

2. An appendectomy incision in a 14-year-old boy that was initially left open because of a ruptured appendix with contamination of the wound. The wound was closed as a delayed primary closure on the 4th postoperative day.

3. A thyroidectomy incision in a 24-year-old woman operated on for a papillary carcinoma.

4. A below-knee amputation stump on a 69-year-old diabetic man with severe peripheral vascular disease.

5. A midline abdominal incision in a cachectic 83-year-old man with carcinomatosis who was operated on for intestinal obstruction.

6. An arm incision for creation of a dialysis fistula in a 56-year-old patient with chronic renal failure.

STUDY QUESTIONS

1 Describe the biological processes involved in the three phases of wound healing.

2 What are some of the conditions, illustrated in the above patients, that can adversely affect wound healing?

3 What factors influence the strength of a healing wound?

4 What can the surgeon do to optimize the healing process?

Common Ambulatory Skin and Soft Tissue Problems

John B. Herrmann, M.D.

REFERENCES

1. *Essentials of General Surgery*—Lawrence: Chapter 11.

2. *Principles of Surgery*—Schwartz: Chapters 14 and 46.

3. *Textbook of Surgery*—Sabiston: Chapters 21 and 45.

4. *Clinical Surgery*—Davis: Chapter 62.

5. *Current Surgical Diagnosis and Treatment*—Way: Chapers 45 and 48.

6. *Essentials of Surgery*—Sabiston: Chapter 37.

Clean Laceration

A 10-year-old boy puts his arm through a glass window while roughhousing with his brother. He sustains a 4-inch laceration of his medial forearm. Bleeding is controlled by pressure using a clean towel. He is brought to your emergency room 20 minutes later, where inspection shows a clean laceration as described with no significant bleeding.

STUDY QUESTIONS

1 Describe your examination of the patient to rule out any significant nerve, tendon, or blood vessel injury.

2 Describe your management of the local wound in a step-by-step fashion from initial cleansing to final dressing.

3 Would you employ any local or systemic antibiotics or other anti-infective agents?

4 Describe your follow-up care of this patient.

5 Outline the phases of wound healing as they pertain to this patient. What are some of the conditions that could impair the healing process?

Dirty Wound

A 27-year-old farm worker is cleaning out the stable when he cuts his leg on a rusty scythe. He applies a crude bandage and continues to work. That evening, 8 hours later, he comes to your emergency room because of pain and throbbing in the leg. On examination he has a 3-inch gash on his leg that is tender and slightly red around the edges.

STUDY QUESTIONS

1 How would you initially manage this wound? Please outline in a step-by-step fashion.

2 Would you consider using any local or systemic antibiotics? Other anti-infective agents?

3 Discuss the differences between primary healing, delayed primary healing, secondary healing, and tertiary healing.

4 How would you manage this wound if it was obviously grossly infected when the patient returned for a checkup 3 days later?

Minor Emergency Ward Cases

Describe your management of each of the following cases, which present to your emergency award during one summer weekend.

a. A knife cut on the hand of a 14-year-old boy.

b. A puncture wound of the foot from a rusty nail in a 6-year-old child.

c. Multiple jagged lacerations of the knuckles in an inebriated factory worker who was involved in a fight at the local tavern when he slugged his adversary in the mouth.

d. A young girl who is bitten on the face by a "friendly" neighborhood dog.

e. Amputation of the pad of the right index finger of a 40-year-old salesman while working in his home workshop.

f. A 9-year-old boy with full-thickness abrasion of his left knee sustained in a fall from his bicycle. There is dirt and gravel embedded in the remaining skin and subcutaneous tissue.

g. An 18-year-old man with a laceration that was sutured 4 days ago and is obviously grossly infected.

h. A 6-year-old girl with a painful subungual hematoma following a crush injury to her right forefinger.

i. A 43-year-old diabetic with an infection under the lateral margin of the fingernail of her right ring finger. The finger is swollen and she cannot remove her ring.

j. A 34-year-old colleague who has developed a very painful infection in the pad of his left thumb following a needle stick.

Minor Surgical Problems in the Office

One afternoon a week you perform a number of minor surgical procedures in your office. Your schedule this afternoon shows the following cases.

a. A 49-year-old woman with a 3 × 2 × 2 cm fatty tumor on her back.

b. A 38-year-old man with a painful ingrown toenail on his right foot. The toenail is thickened and deformed.

c. A 45-year-old woman with a wen of her scalp.

d. A 29-year-old woman with a painful wart on the ball of her left foot.

e. A 69-year-old man with multiple nevi on his back and arms.

STUDY QUESTIONS

1 Discuss your management of each of the above problems, including your techniques of local anesthesia, extent of excision, surgical repair, type of dressing, and postoperative care.

Surgical Infections

John B. Herrmann, M.D.

REFERENCES

1. *Essentials of General Surgery*—Lawrence: Chapter 12.

2. *Principles of Surgery*—Schwartz: Chapter 15.

3. *Textbook of Surgery*—Sabiston: Chapter 14.

4. *Clinical Surgery*—Davis: Chapters 14 and 36.

5. *Current Surgical Diagnosis and Treatment*—Way: Chapter 9.

6. *Essentials of Surgery*—Sabiston: Chapter 11.

7. *Principles of Basic Surgical Practice*—James et al.: Chapter 10.

A Tender Mass in the Thigh

A 56-year-old, insulin-dependent diabetic woman comes to see you in the office with a tender, inflamed 4 × 6 cm fluctuant swelling on her right thigh in the area of her insulin injections. Her temperature is 38°C (101.5°F). Laboratory studies done in the office show a WBC of 12,600 and a blood sugar of 270 mg/100 ml.

STUDY QUESTIONS

1 What is your diagnosis? Distinguish between cellulitis, abscess, furuncle, carbuncle, erysipelas, lymphangitis, and lymphadenitis.

2 How would you confirm your diagnosis?

3 How would you treat this patient?

4 What instruction would you give the patient to avoid a recurrence of this problem?

Postoperative Wound Drainage with Fever

Eighteen hours following a right hemicolectomy for a carcinoma of the cecum, your patient develops a high fever to 40°C (104°F), tachycardia, and delirium. Examination of his abdominal incision reveals tenderness, crepitation, erythema and a watery, brownish sweet smelling drainage from between the sutures.

STUDY QUESTIONS

1 What do you suspect is the diagnosis? How would you confirm It?

2 What is the appropriate treatment of this serious complication?

3 Under what circumstances does a problem like this occur?

4 What are some of the other unusual but serious infections that complicate surgical operations or that require surgical management?

SICU Sepsis

A 76-year-old man underwent an abdominoperineal resection for rectal cancer two days ago. He has been in the intensive care unit with a Swan-Ganz catheter and an arterial line for monitoring purposes. He suddenly develops a shaking chill, a temperature of 39°C (103°F), and a drop in blood pressure to 90/60 mm Hg with a pulse rate of 130 (sinus tachycardia by monitor).

STUDY QUESTIONS

1 What are some of the possible causes of his hypotension? Do you think his fever is related to this event?

2 What further diagnostic studies would you recommend?

3 What initial treatment is indicated?

4 What findings would lead you to change your course of treatment?

Postoperative Fever

Your patient is a 39-year-old woman who underwent an uneventful elective cholecystectomy yesterday. This morning on rounds her temperature is 38.5°C (101.5°F).

STUDY QUESTIONS

1 What are some of the possible causes of her fever? What cause is the most likely one?

2 With your treatment, the patient became afebrile and was doing well until the 5th postoperative day, when she spiked another fever to 38°C (100.4°F). What are the likely causes of fever at this stage postoperatively, and how would you make the diagnosis of each? How would each be treated?

3 Assuming that you find that her incision has become red, tender, swollen, and painful, consistent with a wound infection, how would you treat this complication?

Prophylactic Antibiotic Usage

A 65-year-old man is scheduled for an elective resection of an abdominal aortic aneurysm and replacement with a knitted Dacron bifurcation graft.

STUDY QUESTIONS

1 What is the risk of an infected aortic graft developing in the postoperative period? What are the consequences of such an infection?

2 What steps should be taken to minimize the risk of infection? Should prophylactic antibiotics be used? if so, which antibiotic? What dose? How many doses?

3 Which of the following operations are considered indications for prophylactic antibiotics, and which antibiotics should be used?
(*a*). Acute nonperforated appendicitis;
(*b*). Inguinal hernia repair;
(*c*). Total hip replacement;
(*d*). Cholecystectomy and common bile duct exploration for obstruction;
(*e*). Partial gastrectomy for ulcer;
(*f*). Partial gastrectomy for cancer;
(*g*). Modified radical mastectomy;
(*h*). Lysis of adhesions for intestinal obstruction;
(*i*). Sigmoid resection for diverticulitis;
(*j*). Pneumonectomy for cancer;
(*k*). Mitral valve replacement;
(*l*). Total laryngectomy and radical neck dissection;
(*m*). Parathyroidectomy.

Intraabdominal Abscess

A 42-year-old man underwent an emergency operation for a perforated duodenal ulcer ten days ago. Although he initially appeared to be doing well, he has developed an increasingly febrile course over the past 3 days, with spiking temperatures to 40°C (100.4°F), abdominal distension, and diminished bowel sounds. The abdomen is mildly tender and no masses are felt. An abdominal ultrasound suggests a pelvic and right subhepatic abscess.

STUDY QUESTIONS

1 How would you confirm the diagnosis?

2 What are some of the treatment options? Which one would you suggest?

3 Despite your treatment, the patient remains febrile and on nasogastric suction. What further treatment would you suggest?

<h1>SECTION 8</h1>

Trauma and Burns

Michael D. Wertheimer, M.D.

REFERENCES

1. *Essentials of General Surgery*—Lawrence: Chapter 13.

2. *Principles of Surgery*—Schwartz: Chapters 6 and 7.

3. *Textbook of Surgery*—Sabiston: Chapters 12 and 16.

4. *Clinical Surgery*—Davis: Chapters 69 through 72.

5. *Current Surgical Diagnosis and Treatment*—Way: Chapters 14 and 15.

6. *Essentials of Surgery*—Sabiston: Chapters 9 and 13.

7. *Principles of Basic Surgical Practice*—James et al.: Chapters 40 through 50.

Sledding Accident

An 11-year-old boy is brought to the emergency room 1 hour after a sledding accident in which his sled hit a tree. He is alert and complains only of left flank, abdominal, and chest pain. BP 100/60 mm Hg. P 110. R 24. Physical examination reveals only diffuse left-sided abdominal tenderness and point tenderness over the left lower rib cage in the posterior axillary line.

STAT laboratory studies reveal Hgb 13.6 gm/dl, Hct 35%, and WBC 10,200. Urinalysis is negative except for 10-15 RBC/hpf. Kidney, ureter, bladder (KUB) and chest films show fractures of the left tenth and eleventh ribs. While you are looking at the x-rays, the nurse runs in to tell you that your patient's blood pressure has dropped to 85/50 mm Hg and he is cold and clammy.

STUDY QUESTIONS

1 What do you think has happened?

2 Detail the resuscitative measures you would institute to stabilize the patient.

3 How would you confirm your diagnosis? What are the indications, risks, and accuracy of paracentesis and abdominal CT scans in this setting?

4 What would be your definitive treatment?

5 Are there any alternative forms of treatment?

6 Are there any long-term risks resulting from your treatment?

7 Discuss the possible associated intraabdominal injuries that could occur in such an accident.

8 What are the common postoperative problems seen in the setting of blunt abdominal injury, and what is their treatment?

Multiple Stab Wounds

A 22-year-old man is brought to the emergency room by the police having sustained multiple stab wounds in a street fight. Physical examination reveals a healthy, somewhat inebriated man with BP 120/80 mm Hg, P 80, and R 16. There are stab wounds in the epigastrium, left lower quadrant, right arm, and right shoulder without significant bleeding. The abdomen is soft and mildly tender in the area of the wounds. Bowel sounds are hypoactive.

Laboratory data show Hgb 14.9 gm/dl, Hct 42%, WBC 11,500, and normal urinalysis. Plain abdominal and chest radiographs are unremarkable.

STUDY QUESTIONS

1 What further diagnostic studies might be indicated in this patient?

2 How would you initially manage this patient?

3 What is the definitive treatment of a penetrating abdominal injury?

4 Discuss the treatment of penetrating injuries of the stomach, small bowel, colon, liver, and pancreas.

5 Would management be any different if these were gunshot injuries?

6 How would you manage the other soft tissues injuries?

Massive Blunt Trauma

A 38-year-old cement truck driver lost control of his vehicle on a steep grade. The truck slammed into an embankment and rolled over on its side, pinning the driver in the cab. The helicopter trauma team arrived with the police, and after a prolonged extrication (60 minutes) the patient was stabilized on the scene. Endotracheal intubation and venous access were achieved, and he was stabilized on a backboard. The patient was unconscious, blood pressure was 40/0 mm Hg, and he had no spontaneous respiration or extremity movement. He was transferred in 13 minutes to the trauma center, where you and the hospital trauma team are waiting to receive him.

STUDY QUESTIONS

1 Who are the members of your trauma team; what tasks have you assigned each individual, and what are the first five priorities to attend to in this patient's initial resuscitation and primary evaluation survey?

2 What are the ABCs of effective resuscitation? What is the primary survey?

3 What are the specifics of initial fluid resuscitation?

4 What is the secondary survey? How is the neurologic assessment made, and what is the Glasgow Coma Scale?

5 What is this patient's trauma score and what does that predict about the patient's prognosis for survival?

6 What is the role of paracentesis in the unconscious patient? Of head and body CT scans?

7 What laboratory and radiographic studies are urgently needed (in order of priority) in this patient's first few minutes in the emergency room?

8 What laboratory tests and x-rays are of secondary importance?

9 How does one establish priorities of injury, orchestrate the workup, and expeditiously institute therapy? What is the ''Golden Hour'' for the multiply injured trauma patient?

The patient is a 45-year-old man who was brought into the emergency room unconscious. He was brought in by ambulance after an apparent head-on collision in which he was the driver. There is no other history.

Physical examination: BP 40/0 mm Hg, P 40, R 60. General: cyanotic and unconscious. Respiration: trachea midline, very shallow respirations, no resonance to percussion, multiple bilateral palpable rib fractures, questionable paradoxical respirations.

STUDY QUESTIONS

1 How sick is this man on a scale of 1 to 10 (10 being the sickest)?

2 What system is primarily deranged?

3 What emergency measures would you take, and in what order?

4 If you have treated his primary problem correctly, he is more stable but his blood pressure is still 80/40 mm Hg and pulse is 120.

   a. What are your possible diagnoses as a cause of his hypotension?

   b. How would you evaluate your three most likely diagnoses?

   c. How would you treat them?

Head-on Collision 2

Assume that we are now treating a patient that has an identical history to the patient in the preceding case (8-4). However, his physical examination shows the following: BP 40/O mm Hg, P 40, R 60. General: cyanotic and unresponsive. Respiration: trachea shift to the right, absent breath sounds on the left, hyperresonance to percussion on the left. CV: decreased heart sounds, neck veins distended.

STUDY QUESTIONS

1 You have only a few seconds to make a diagnosis and initiate therapy.

   a. Diagnosis?

   b. Emergency treatment?

2 If you did the correct thing, the patient is alive (but not well). If you did not do the correct thing, call the Medical Examiner. Assuming the former, you now reassess him and find: BP 100/50 mm Hg, P 120, R 30. He is awake, his hematocrit has dropped from 40 to 30% in one hour, and his chest x-ray shows a left pleural effusion.

   a. What is happening?

   b. How would you treat him next? Why or why not use each of the following interventions? 1. Thoracentesis; 2. Give blood; 3. Don't give blood; 4. Operate; 5. Chest tube.

   c. If you decided against operation, when would you operate on such a patient?

3 You have treated the above and now find the following: BP 100/50 mm Hg, CVP 25, P 130.

   a. What is your conclusion now?

   b. How would you confirm it?

   c. How would you treat this?

Gunshot Wound

The patient is a 68-year-old farmer who suddenly experienced left chest pain prior to coming to the hospital.

He was tending his cows during deer hunting season when he felt a blow to his left chest and simultaneously heard a gunshot. He fell to the ground and was brought to the emergency room with dyspnea.

Physical examination: BP 100/50 mm Hg, P 120, R 40. General: cyanotic. Chest: sucking wound left chest, tympany to percussion of left, decreased breath sounds left. Abdomen: nontender, no masses or wounds.

STUDY QUESTIONS

1 What treatment do you initiate as the first step?

2 Why?

3 What is the pathophysiology of a "sucking" chest wound?

4 What is the difference between an open, closed, and tension pneumothorax?

5 Do you think the patient will require an operation? How would you decide if he will?

Penetrating Vascular Injury

A 43-year-old lawyer and his 16-year-old son are clearing off the badly overgrown yard of their newly acquired summer cottage. The man is cutting down large bushes with a chain saw, while the son is mowing the grass and weeds with a long scythe. Inadvertently they get too close to each other. At the end of a long sweeping motion, the tip of the scythe pierces the upper inner aspect of the man's thigh. There is profuse hemorrhage, which the boy finally staunches with a crude tourniquet made from his T-shirt and belt. They arrive in your emergency room 25 minutes later. When the tourniquet is removed, there is no more bleeding. The foot appears normal, and there is a palpable dorsalis pedis pulse.

STUDY QUESTIONS

1 What do you suspect is the nature of the injury? Why has the bleeding stopped?

2 What is the best way to control superficial hemorrhage? Deeper hemorrhage in the extremities? The abdomen? The chest? The skull?

3 What are the hazards of tourniquets?

4 Does this patient require any further evaluation or treatment, since the bleeding has stopped and circulation appears adequate?

5 What are the possible early and late sequelae of untreated vascular injuries?

6 What is the natural history of a traumatic false aneurysm? A traumatic A-V fistula?

7 What nonpenetrating injuries can cause major vascular damage? How is the diagnosis made?

Blunt Vascular Injury

While picking apples, a 12-year-old boy falls out of a tree, landing on his right upper arm. He arrives at the emergency room with pain, crepitus, swelling, and abnormal mobility of the midhumeral region. His hand is pale, cool, and pulseless.

STUDY QUESTIONS

1 What do you suspect is the nature of the injury?

2 What physical findings are useful in evaluating arterial injury? What findings indicate threatened tissue survival due to ischemia?

3 What further diagnostic studies might be useful?

4 What treatment would be indicated for extravascular compression by bone fragments or hematoma? Arterial laceration? Arterial thrombosis?

5 What are early and late sequelae of severe ischemia? What is Volkmann's contracture?

6 What other orthopaedic injuries are sometimes associated with vascular injuries?

Thermal Burn

A 47-year-old hunter is transferred to your hospital approximately 6 hours after an accident in which his flannel shirt caught fire while he was lighting a kerosene stove in a hunting camp. His companions put out the fire but not before he sustained burns over the area of his body covered by his long-sleeved shirt, as well as some injury to his hands and face. He was taken to a local, small community hospital by his friends and was immediately transferred to your hospital by ambulance.

Upon arrival at your hospital the patient was agitated and slightly confused with a blood pressure of 90/60 mm Hg and a pulse of 130. The extent of the burn injury was as described above. There was no history of any other medical problem.

STUDY QUESTIONS

1 List step-by-step the diagnostic and therapeutic procedures indicated in the early management of this patient.

2 Using the "Rule of Nines" calculate the approximate percentage of body surface area burn.

3 Describe the pathological classification of burn depth and the clinical significance of burn depth. What clinical findings are used to estimate burn depth? What depth of burn would you expect to predominate in your patient?

4 Assuming that the patient weighs 80 kg, calculate the estimated fluid requirements for this patient: (a) In the next 2 hours; (b) In the following 16 hours; (c) In the second 24 hours.

5 How would you monitor fluid therapy?

6 How would you manage the burn wound?

7 Discuss the prevention and management of sepsis in the burn patient.

8 What are the nutritional requirements in this patient? How are you going to manage his nutritional support?

9 Describe the composition of the medical care team needed for the care of this patient.

10 In contrast to this complicated case, how would you manage a minor (less than 5% body surface area) burn?

11 What are the differences between a thermal burn, an electrical burn, a chemical burn, and a radiation burn?

12 Discuss the modifications of management necessary to care for large numbers of burns that might occur in a disaster.

Electrical Burn

A 46-year-old construction worker drove his underground tractor across a high-tension wire of 35,000–40,000 volts, sustaining electrical burns to both hands and arms, with the point of exit in the back of both calves. He did not lose consciousness and was brought to the emergency room with stable vital signs. General examination of the patient showed an area of dry eschar extending from the tips of the fingers to the elbow and pain and swelling of both right and left hand and forearm. No pulse was palpable on the left side; however, the patient complained of anesthesia in the distribution of the median nerve. A Foley catheter inserted recovered 150 ml of blood-tinged urine.

STUDY QUESTIONS

1 Describe the pathogenesis of electrical burns with respect to the following:
   (a) The voltage of the current;
   (b) The intensity or amperage;
   (c) Distance at the point of contact;
   (d) The resistance at the point of grounding;
   (e) Duration of contact;
   (f) Pathway of the current through the body; and
   (g) The type of current.

2 What is the range of temperature generated by the electrical arcing in high-voltage injuries?

3 Contrast the relationship of the type of tissue, its resistance to electrical current, and the degree of thermal damage.

4 List the indications and necessity of escharotomies and fasciotomies.

5 Describe the relationship of electrical injuries to clostridial infection and the need for anticlostridial prophylaxis.

6 Describe the relationship of the type of electrical burn with respect to the surgical management.

Chemical Burn

A worker in a glass etching factory was brought to the emergency room after he came in contact with hydrofluoric acid to his left dominant hand involving the palm and the dorsum of the hand. The liquid also splashed on areas of the lower abdomen and the interior aspect of the left thigh.

STUDY QUESTIONS

1 What is the initial emergency room management of a chemical burn caused by hydrofluoric acid?

2 What kinds of dressings are used after initial treatment; how frequently are they changed; and are any tropical agents used with the dressing changes?

3 Is any debridement, excision, grafting, or topical chemotherapy indicated in chemical burns?

4 Describe changes in management if the injury were due to sulfuric acid, sodium hydroxide, and phosphorus.

Frostbite

A 59-year-old man was brought into the emergency room after he was found by the police wandering around in the snow without shoes or socks. The patient was somewhat inebriated and on examination was found to have frostbite injuries to both feet and legs to the level of the knees.

STUDY QUESTIONS

1 Review the acute treatment of frostbite injuries.

2 Discuss the use of low-molecular-weight dextran or heparin.

3 Discuss the role of regional sympathetic nerve block.

4 Discuss the role of rapid warming.

5 Discuss the role and timing of surgical treatment.

Radiation Injury

A 22-year-old laboratory technician is seen in the emergency room shortly after she was exposed to ionizing radiation to the dorsa of both hands while working with a faulty x-ray machine. On examination both hands appear to be normal except for slight erythema.

STUDY QUESTIONS

1 What are the different types of radiation?

2 How is the wavelength of the radiation related to the degree of injury?

3 List in decreasing order wavelengths in the electromagnetic spectrum.

4 Describe the timing of symptoms of acute radiation with respect to infrared radiation, ultraviolet radiation, and x-ray radiation.

5 Describe the clinical symptoms of x-ray radiation injury to the skin within 7 to 10 days of injury.

6 Describe the signs and symptoms of chronic radiation injury.

7 Discuss secondary ulceration, osteoradionecrosis, and malignant changes.

8 What is the role of solar protective agents in the treatment of radiodermatitis?

Abdominal Wall

John B. Herrmann, M.D.

REFERENCES

1. *Essentials of General Surgery*—Lawrence: Chapter 14.
2. *Principles of Surgery*—Schwartz: Chapter 35.
3. *Textbook of Surgery*—Sabiston: Chapters 28 and 38.
4. *Clinical Surgery*—Davis: Chapter 51.
5. *Current Surgical Diagnosis and Treatment*—Way: Chapter 34.
6. *Essentials of Surgery*—Sabiston: Chapter 32.
7. *Principles of Basic Surgical Practice*—James et al.: Chapter 25.

A Bulge in the Groin

A 60-year-old obese man presents with complaints of mild discomfort and a bulge in his groin for the past 3 months.

STUDY QUESTIONS

1 What are the specific questions to ask this patient relative to his family, social, and past medical history, and review of systems?

2 What are the predisposing factors in the formation of an inguinal hernia in a patient of this age? How would you diagnose and treat these conditions?

3 Discuss groin hernias and differentiate them one from another regarding their distribution in the population.

4 What is the differential diagnosis of a groin mass?

5 List the anatomic structures encountered in the repair of an inguinal hernia. The first structure encountered is skin.

A Painful Groin Mass with Vomiting

A 35-year-old man is seen by you in the emergency room with a 6-hour history of a painful right groin mass accompanied by crampy abdominal pain, nausea, and vomiting. He has a history of a bulge in his groin following an episode of pain while lifting a heavy bag of cement several years ago. The bulge usually disappeared when he lay down.

Physical examination shows a tender soft mass in the right groin with hyperactive bowel sounds. Vital signs are BP 120/70 mm Hg, P 90, R 15, T 37°C (98.6°F). Laboratory studies are normal. Abdominal x-ray shows dilated loops of small bowel.

STUDY QUESTIONS

1 What is your tentative diagnosis?

2 Would you recommend any further tests?

3 Describe your proposed treatment step by step.

4 Differentiate between reducible, incarcerated, and strangulated hernia. What influence does this have on the diagnosis?

5 Describe the relative risks of complications in each of the several types of groin hernias.

6 At operation, a "sliding" inguinal hernia is discovered. Describe the anatomy of this entity and the method of repair.

An Umbilical Bulge

A 1-month-old infant is brought to your office because of a bulge in the belly button. Your examination reveals this bulge to be 1 1/2 cm in diameter.

STUDY QUESTIONS

1 What would you advise the parents?

2 How should a similar bulge in an adult be managed?

3 What might be the etiology of such a bulge in the adult patient?

4 List the various types of abdominal wall hernias and discuss their management.

Abdominal Wall Defect in a Newborn

A newborn infant is noted to have a protrusion of bowel through a defect in the umbilical area at the time of birth.

STUDY QUESTIONS

1 Distinguish between omphalocele and gastroschisis.

2 Discuss the management of each.

3 What are the possible accompanying conditions?

4 What are the complications of management of these conditions?

5 What is the prognosis?

<hr>

Incisional Hernia

An obese 75-year-old woman is referred to you with an enormous bulge in her abdominal wall in the area of an old paramedian abdominal incision. She had had a left hemicolectomy for colon cancer 10 years previously, and had a postoperative wound infection at that time. The bulging at the incision has been progressive, although it disappears when she lies down.

STUDY QUESTIONS

1 What is the likely diagnosis?

2 Give the indications for nonsurgical and surgical management.

3 Assuming this is a complication of her previous operation, how could it have been avoided? What are other predisposing factors?

4 Discuss the principles of surgical repair.

5 What is the incidence of recurrence?

Esophagus

John B. Herrmann, M.D.

REFERENCES

1. *Essentials of General Surgery*—Lawrence: Chapter 15.

2. *Principles of Surgery*—Schwartz: Chapter 25.

3. *Textbook of Surgery*—Sabiston: Chapter 27.

4. *Clinical Surgery*—Davis: Chapter 43.

5. *Current Surgical Diagnosis and Treatment*—Way: Chapter 21.

6. *Essentials of Surgery*—Sabiston: Chapter 21.

7. *Principles of Basic Surgical Practice*—James et al.: Chapter 17.

Nocturnal Regurgitation and Dysphagia

A 76-year-old man complains of episodes of regurgitation of food into his mouth at night with bouts of coughing. He has also noted mild difficulty in swallowing, with a sensation of fullness in his throat.

STUDY QUESTIONS

1 What is your preliminary diagnosis?

2 How would you confirm your diagnostic impression?

3 What is the etiology of this condition?

4 What type of treatment would you recommend?

5 Do lesions of this type occur at other levels of the esophagus? Is the etiology similar? Is the treatment the same?

Progressive Dysphagia

Your patient is a 55-year-old man who has had difficulty in swallowing for 4 months. This has been progressively more severe, and while it initially occurred only with solids, it now occurs with liquids also. During this same time, he has had a 15-pound weight loss but no other GI or pulmonary symptoms. On close questioning, he thinks the food sticks in the lower part of his chest.

Physical examination is negative except for slight emaciation. The liver is normal, the stool guaiac is trace positive.

STUDY QUESTIONS

1 What are some of the possible diagnoses? Rank them in decreasing order of likelihood.

2 Which two studies are mandatory in establishing a diagnosis? In what order should they be performed?

3 How would you treat your first, second, and third diagnoses (from your answer to question 1)?

4 If this is a tumor, what cell type or types is it likely to be? Would you do a liver scan? Would it alter your therapy for the tumor?

5 If this is a stricture, what are the possible causes of it?

6 Are there any nonobstructive causes of difficulty in swallowing? What are they?

Chronic Dysphagia

A 48-year-old man presents with a long history of progressive dysphagia, nighttime regurgitation with bouts of coughing, and substernal discomfort on swallowing. A barium swallow shows a dilated, nonperistaltic esophagus with a "bird beak" narrowing of the esophagogastric junction.

STUDY QUESTIONS

1 What is the most likely diagnosis? What other conditions should be considered?

2 What further diagnostic tests would you suggest?

3 What is the etiology of the most likely diagnosis?

4 Discuss the various modalities of treatment available. What would you recommend?

5 Discuss the indications for surgical treatment of this condition. What operations are available?

Heartburn

A 56-year-old, moderately obese woman comes to your office complaining of increasingly severe heartburn over the past few months. In the past, this has been occasional and relieved by antacid. Her symptoms are now more persistent, less easily relieved, and accompanied by pain on swelling.

STUDY QUESTIONS

1 Her symptoms are typical of what condition?

2 How would you confirm the diagnosis?

3 What is the etiology of this condition?

4 What are the potential complications if this condition remains untreated?

5 What would you recommend for initial treatment? What if initial treatment is unsuccessful?

6 What is the relationship between this condition and a sliding hiatal hernia? A paraesophageal hernia? What is the treatment of each?

Stomach and Duodenum

John B. Herrmann, M.D., and Micheal D. Wertheimer, M.D.

REFERENCES

1. *Essentials of General Surgery*—Lawrence: Chapter 16.

2. *Principles of Surgery*—Schwartz: Chapter 28.

3. *Textbook of Surgery*—Sabiston: Chapters 30 and 31.

4. *Clinical Surgery*—Davis: Chapter 44.

5. *Current Surgical Diagnosis and Treatment*—Way: Chapter 24.

6. *Essentials of Surgery*—Sabiston: Chapter 23.

7. *Principles of Basic Surgical Practice*—James et al.: Chapter 22.

Heartburn and Epigastric Pain

A 46-year-old investment banker consults you because of persistent heartburn and epigastric pain. He works 16-hour days, frequently misses meals, smokes 2 packs of cigarettes per day, and makes insider deals at multiple-martini lunches. He sometimes is awakened by pain but denies nausea, vomiting, blood in the stool, or weight loss. His last physical examination was 6 years ago, and he wants an expeditious and direct solution to his problem.

STUDY QUESTIONS

1 Peptic ulcer is your working diagnosis; what can you say about the natural history, epidemiology, and pathogenesis of peptic ulcer disease as it pertains to this patient? Are there risk factors?

2 Compare and contrast the indications for and value of each of the following diagnostic studies in patients with suspected gastric or duodenal ulcer disease: upper gastrointestinal roentgenograms, endoscopy with biopsy, gastric analysis, serum gastrin levels, and the secretin stimulation test. What single test do you recommend to this patient?

3 What is the value of the history in such patients? Is it reasonable to begin treatment without a diagnostic workup based solely on the history?

4 Described in detail the nonoperative management of peptic ulcer disease, including antacids, H_2 blockers, surface coating agents, diet, and reversible life style risk factors.

5 What are the complications of peptic ulcer disease? Their surgical management?

6 Define intractability in peptide ulcer patients. What is your approach to the complex psychosocial and physiological circumstances in this patient whose symptoms persist or recur after initial treatment?

7 What are the indications for surgical intervention electively for intractable peptic ulcer disease?

8 Draw and describe the common operations performed for duodenal ulcer disease, and give the physiologic basis, risks, complications, and results of each.

9 What are the common side effects and physiologic aberrations that may result from operations performed for the treatment of peptic ulcer disease? How frequently do they occur? How are they treated?

Gastric Tumor

A 54-year-old businessman presents with a 3-week history of dysphagia, anorexia and early satiety, and a 10-pound weight loss. Examination in the office reveals a well-developed, somewhat pale middle-aged man in no acute distress. There is mild epigastric tenderness but no palpable masses, and no hepatomegaly.

Two years ago, the patient was admitted with an acute myocardial infarction and underwent coronary artery bypass grafting on an urgent basis. He did well subsequently, but 3 months postoperatively he was found to have a lesser curvature gastric ulcer measuring approximately 1.2 cm in diameter. He was treated with H_2 blockers, antacids, and diet, and a repeat upper GI series 3 months later showed complete healing of the ulcer. He had no further gastrointestinal symptoms until 3 weeks ago.

An upper GI series is performed and shows a large filling defect occupying almost all of the lesser curvature of the stomach; there is partial obstruction at the esophagogastric junction. His hemoglobin is 10.5 gm/dl, hematocrit is 32%, and stool is guaiac positive. He is admitted to the hospital, and the following day has upper GI panendoscopy, which reveals a huge fungating mass occupying the entire lesser curvature. Biopsies show adenocarcinoma.

STUDY QUESTIONS

1 What is considered current good practice in the office management of gastric ulcers? Do you think the patient might have had a different outcome?

2 What further workup would be appropriate in this patient after the diagnosis is made? Should a surgical consultation be obtained?

3 Discuss gastric cancer in terms of its incidence, its epidemiology, and its pathological variants.

4 Discuss signs and symptoms of gastric malignancies and diagnostic manuevers necessary to establish a diagnosis.

FURTHER INFORMATION

The patient is explored in the operating room and found to have an extensive mass involving the entire lesser curvature, celiac plexus, omentum and paraaortic fascia. The liver is grossly free of metastatic disease, but the mass lesion is directly invading the head of the pancreas and abutting the common bile duct.

STUDY QUESTIONS

5 Do you think this patient has a curable cancer? Discuss the results of surgery in gastric malignancy. Are any patients cured of this tumor without an operation?

6 What are the general principles of curative and palliative surgical procedures for patients with gastric neoplasm? What should be done for this patient? Discuss various forms of "palliative gastric resection" and other palliative operations for this disease. How does one reestablish gastrointestinal continuity?

7 What is the role of radiotherapy or chemotherapy in this disease? Intraoperative radiotherapy?

8 Classify other tumors of the distal esophagus and stomach and discuss diagnosis and treatment.

9 What postoperative complications will you anticipate, and what forms of nutritional support might you provide this patient postoperatively?

10 Discuss the nutritional consequences of partial and total gastric resection, and how you would instruct this patient to handle his diet in the office.

Acute Abdominal Pain

A 46-year-old businessman is brought to the emergency room with the sudden onset of severe generalized abdominal pain occurring one half hour previously. Vital signs are: BP 100/60 mm Hg, P 120, and R 28. He is pale and sweaty with a rigid, tender abdomen and no bowel sounds.

STUDY QUESTIONS

1 List your tentative differential diagnosis and how you would proceed to arrive at a correct diagnosis.

2 Discuss your initial resuscitative treatment of this patient. What are you trying to accomplish, and how can you measure the effectiveness of your efforts?

3 Assuming that x-ray examination shows free air under the diaphragm and initial resuscitation has been successful, what further treatment would you recommend? Are there any alternatives? Described them.

4 What are the common and uncommon causes of free air in the abdominal cavity?

5 Assuming that free air was not present, what other surgical and non-surgical conditions could cause this clinical picture?

Upper Gastrointestinal Bleeding

A 54-year-old housewife with a long history of duodenal ulcer disease is admitted to the emergency ward with hematemesis, melana, and collapse. Vital signs are: BP 60/? mm Hg, P 160 and thready, and R 30. Abdomen is soft with mild epigastric tenderness and active bowel sounds. Rectal examination shows tarry guaiac 4+ stool.

STUDY QUESTIONS

1 What is your tentative diagnosis? What are the common causes of massive upper GI bleeding?

2 List your initial resuscitative efforts. How can you monitor their effectiveness?

3 How would you confirm or establish the correct diagnosis?

4 List the indications for surgical intervention in each of the common causes of massive upper GI bleeding.

5 Discuss the appropriate surgical procedure for each of the above diagnoses.

6 List the potential complications of each of the above operations.

Gastric Outlet Obstruction

A 75-year-old patient presents with a 10-day history of vomiting almost everything that he has eaten or drunk. He appears weak, dehydrated, and moderately ill. The abdomen is soft and scaphoid with normal bowel sounds and no palpable masses. Rectal examination is negative with no stool in the ampulla. An upper GI series shows a dilated stomach with only a trickle of barium passing through a deformed duodenal bulb. Laboratory studies show: Hct 56%, WBC 7.500, Na 130 mEq/liter, K 2.0 mEq/liter, Cl 79 mEq/liter, and HCO_3 35 mEq/liter. Arterial blood gases show a pH of 7.50, PCO_2 44 mm Hg, and PO_2 98 mm Hg. Blood urea nitrogen (BUN) is 42 mg/dl.

STUDY QUESTIONS

1 What is your tentative diagnosis?

2 Explain the patient's abnormal electrolytes and acid-base balance.

3 Discuss your initial treatment.

4 Discuss the definitive treatment for this condition.

Small Intestine and Appendix

John B. Herrmann, M.D.

REFERENCES

1. *Essentials of General Surgery*—Lawrence: Chapter 4.

2. *Principles of Surgery*—Schwartz: Chapters 27 and 29.

3. *Textbook of Surgery*—Sabiston: Chapter 32.

4. *Clinical Surgery*—Davis: Chapters 45 and 47.

5. *Current Surgical Diagnosis and Treatment*—Way: Chapters 30 and 31.

6. *Essentials of Surgery*—Sabiston: Chapters 24 and 25.

7. *Principles of Basic Surgical Practice*—James et al.: Chapters 18 and 23.

Crampy Abdominal Pain and Diarrhea

A 22-year-old female patient presents with increasing crampy abdominal pain, weight loss, distention, and intermittent diarrhea. She had a diagnosis of Crohn's disease made 1 year ago on the basis of typical radiologic findings by barium enema, and was placed on sulfa drugs and prednisone, 20 mg per day, at that time.

Physical examination reveals a moderately distended tympanitic abdomen with hyperactive bowel sounds. Liquid feces are present in the rectal ampulla and are guaiac positive. Hematocrit is 30%. The remainder of routine laboratory studies is normal. A barium enema shows increased narrowing of the terminal ileum with proximal bowel distention.

STUDY QUESTIONS

1 What is the most likely cause of her increasing symptoms?

2 Are any further diagnostic studies indicated?

3 What are the options available for treatment at this stage of the disease? What do you think is the best course of treatment?

4 What are the potential complications of each of the possible therapeutic alternatives suggested above? How would you manage them?

5 What is her long-term prognosis?

Abdominal Pain in an Adolescent Girl

A 15-year-old girl comes to the emergency ward with a 36-hour history of abdominal pain, nausea, and anorexia. She was well until early yesterday morning when she was awakened with vague abdominal pain and nausea, but no vomiting. She was unable to eat all day but managed some fluids. The pain, which was initially generalized, has settled in her lower abdomen on the right and become more intense. After an initial bowel movement yesterday morning she has had no further passage of feces or flatus. Having not improved after a restless night, her mother brought her in after finding a temperature of 38.1°C (100.6°F).

On physical examination you confirm a temperature of 38.4°C (101°F), a blood pressure of 110/60 mm Hg, and a pulse of 110. The child looks sick with lower abdominal tenderness, guarding, and rebound tenderness to the right lower quadrant. Bowel sounds are absent and rectal examination shows tenderness in the right pelvic vault. Despite being fairly sexually mature, the girl denies sexual contact. Her last menstrual period was two weeks ago.

STUDY QUESTIONS

1 On the basis of the history and physical findings described above, what is the most likely diagnosis? What are other possible causes of these symptoms and signs?

2 What laboratory studies would you order? What results would you expect? What if the results did not confirm your initial diagnostic impression?

3 What radiologic studies might be helpful in the diagnosis or management of this patient?

4 Describe the pathophysiology of localized abdominal pain, tenderness, rebound tenderness, and spasm. Why are bowel sounds absent?

5 What gynecologic conditions can cause symptoms similar to those described? How would you confirm one of these conditions?

6 Discuss the plan of management for this patient. Write your admission orders.

7 Discuss the indications for surgical intervention. What procedure would you recommend for each of the possible diagnoses?

8 List the potential complications of the more common possible conditions and the management of each.

9 What is the role of antibiotic therapy in the various diagnostic possibilities suggested here?

Abdominal Pain, Vomiting, and Obstipation

A 43-year-old, thin married woman with four children is brought to the emergency department by ambulance with a 48-hour history of crampy abdominal pain, nausea, vomiting, and abdominal distention. Her last bowel movement was yesterday morning. During the past several months she has noted intermittent abdominal cramps with some diarrhea, anorexia, and a 10-pound weight loss. Her past history is negative except for an appendectomy at age 11. In the emergency department, you are asked to examine her.

STUDY QUESTIONS

1 What specific findings must you look for? Describe the expected findings.

2 What specific studies would you order immediately? Name only the specific ones that will assist in confirming the diagnosis and managing the patient.

3 List the various conditions that could cause the symptoms and signs illustrated by this case. List them in order of probability. What are some of the historical details or physical findings that would suggest a specific diagnosis?

4 For each of the possible diagnoses, indicate what, if any, specific studies could be obtained to confirm or rule out the proposed diagnosis. What specific findings would suggest intestinal strangulation?

5 Differentiate between paralytic and mechanical ileus.

6 Describe the fluid and electrolyte changes that commonly occur in this condition.

7 Write the initial intravenous fluid orders for this patient.

8 What additional steps in management are indicated for this patient?

9 For each of the possible diagnoses listed in question 3 above, indicate the optimal specific treatment.

Obstructing Small Bowel Tumor

Your patient, a 36-year-old woman, was found to have gallstones during an evaluation for vague abdominal discomfort, and cholecystectomy was recommended. During the operation a mass was found in the distal ileum with mild dilatation of the proximal small bowel and enlarged lymph nodes palpable at the root of the mesentery. The surgeon asks you to come to the operating room to consult with him on the proper management of your patient.

STUDY QUESTIONS

1 What would you advise on the basis of the above information? Are there any additional questions you would ask?

2 What are the most frequent tumors found in the small intestine? Are there any nonneoplastic lesions that could give the picture described above?

3 What is the preferred management of each of the conditions you have identified in question 2 above? Are some of these conditions best managed medically? How? Discuss the role of surgical resection, radiation therapy, and chemotherapy in the management of neoplasms of the small bowel.

Post-Appendectomy Obstruction

An 18-year-old male is admitted to the emergency room with a 24-hour history of lower abdominal pain, nausea, and vomiting. Acute appendicitis is diagnosed, and a ruptured appendix with early periapendiceal abscess is found at surgery. He undergoes an uneventful appendectomy with drainage. His postoperative course is somewhat stormy but eventually he is discharged on the 10th postoperative day.

Six weeks following the operation he develops crampy abdominal pain with distention, nausea, and vomiting. He had not moved his bowels for 3 days. When seen in the office, his temperature was 37.8°C (100°F). His abdomen was distended and tympanitic. There was mild tenderness periumbilically but no guarding or rebound. There were high-pitched bowel sounds. Rectal examination showed no stool in the ampulla.

Hemoglobin is 16 gm/dl, Hct 48%, WBC 11,600, differential normal. Six weeks ago upon discharge they were 13 gm/dl and 38%. Serum electrolytes are normal; blood urea nitrogen (BUN) is 28 mg/dl, creatinine 1.2 mg/dl, sugar 106 mg/100 ml. X-ray of the abdomen in upright and supine views show multiple dilated loops of small bowel, with numerous air-fluid levels. There is no gas or stool visible in the colon.

The patient is admitted to the hospital.

STUDY QUESTIONS

1 What is the most likely diagnosis? Do you think his condition can be cured without an operation? What is the initial plan of management?

2 If a conservative plan of management is elected, how do you know if he is improving or if he continues to be obstructed? What form of gastrointestinal decompression would you use in this patient? How long a trial of conservative management would you try?

3 What are the indications for early operative intervention in postoperative acute small bowel obstruction?

4 Define and differentiate bowel obstruction and paralytic ileus.

5 Characterize three main categories of mechanical obstruction and list three samples of each.

6 Characterize the fluid ambulance that accompanies distal small bowel obstruction (e.g., why are serum electrolytes usually normal?) and outline the essentials of preoperative management.

7 If a resection of the small intestine is required at operation, describe the various techniques available for reestablishing gastrointestinal continuity. For an obstructed small bowel, why do you think surgeons usually favor side-to-side techniques?

8 If one encounters gangrenous small bowel, sometimes a "second look" operation is performed; do you know what this is and why it is considered?

9 After small bowel resection, would you advise early postoperative feeding via the enteral route? What are other methods of maintaining nutrition following small bowel resection?

10 Outline where differential absorption of minerals and nutrients occurs in the small bowel. Detail what derangements of digestion and absorption can be anticipated when the terminal ileum is resected.

A Child with Rectal Bleeding

A 4-year-old boy is brought to the emergency room because of the passage of a grossly bloody bowel movement noted by his mother. Vital signs are stable. Abdominal and rectal examinations are negative, but maroon-colored blood is present in the ampulla. Hematocrit is 36%.

STUDY QUESTIONS

1 List the possible causes of GI bleeding in this patient.

2 What further diagnostic studies are indicated to localize the source of bleeding and determine its etiology?

3 Assuming no source can be found in the colon or stomach-duodenum by appropriate studies, what would be the most likely source of bleeding from the small bowel?

4 How can this diagnosis be confirmed, and what is the indicated treatment?

Acute Abdomen

A 14-year-old boy is seen by you in the emergency room at 6:00 PM. with a 12-hour history of abdominal pain. He awoke at 6:00 AM. this morning with a vague stomach ache and did not feel like eating his usual hearty breakfast. His mother kept him home from school and he stayed in bed most of the day. He had a normal bowel movement yesterday, but was unable to move his bowels today, despite the urge to defecate. This morning he was nauseated and vomited on one occasion, but this has improved. This afternoon he complained of more severe pain on the right side of his abdomen, and his mother noted an elevation of his temperature to 38.7°C (100.6°F) orally.

Examination reveals a well-developed adolescent boy who appears moderately ill. Temperature is 38.4°C (101.1°F) per rectum. Abdominal examination reveals moderate tenderness, maximum on the right side of the abdomen and in the right flank. There is no spasm or point tenderness, and mild cough and rebound tenderness referred to the right. Bowel sounds are present but hypoactive. Rectal examination is negative.

Laboratory findings show a hemoglobin of 16.1 gm/dl and hematocrit of 48%. WBC is 12,500 with 50 segs, 27 bands, 15 lymphocytes, six monocytes, one eosinophil, and one basophil. Urinalysis is normal except for 10–15 WBCs and 5–10 RBCs per high power field.

STUDY QUESTIONS

1 What is the most likely diagnosis?

2 What other diagnoses should be considered?

3 Are there any atypical findings in this case? Can they be explained?

4 Are there any further diagnostic tests that should be done?

5 How would you manage this patient?

6 Are there alternatives to your proposed treatment?

7 What are some of the other causes of acute abdominal pain? Do all of these entities require a surgical approach?

8 Outline your approach to the evaluation and management of a patient with acute abdominal pain.

Colon and Rectum

Michael D. Wertheimer, M.D.

REFERENCES

1. *Essentials of General Surgery*—Lawrence: Chapter 5.

2. *Principles of Surgery*—Schwartz: Chapter 28.

3. *Textbook of Surgery*—Sabiston: Chapter 3.

4. *Clinical Surgery*—Davis: Chapter 46.

5. *Current Surgical Diagnosis and Treatment*—Way: Chapters 32 and 33.

6. *Essentials of Surgery*—Sabiston: Chapter 26.

7. *Principles of Basic Surgical Practice*—James et al.: Chapter 24.

Rectal Bleeding

A 66-year-old man is seen in the office with a 3-week history of intermittent rectal bleeding. There has been no change in bowel habits and no weight loss or other constitutional symptoms. The bleeding is mild and intermittent, is dark red, and usually occurs just after his bowel movements. There is no diarrhea or mucus in the stool.

Examination in the office is essentially unremarkable. Rectal examination shows no palpable masses; stool is 3+ guaiac positive. There are no abdominal masses and no tenderness.

STUDY QUESTIONS

1 What diagnostic steps should be taken in the workup of this patient? Should he be admitted immediately to the hospital:

2 What is the differential diagnosis of rectal bleeding in an adult?

FURTHER INFORMATION

The patient undergoes proctosigmoidoscopy in your office and you are able to advance the scope easily to 25 cm. No polyps, diverticula, or tumor are visualized. The mucosa shows no significant abnormalities. On removal of the instrument, prominent internal hemorrhoids are visualized. A barium enema is done: numerous diverticula are noted throughout the sigmoid and descending colon. An area of spasm is noted at the proximal sigmoid loop; it does not distend well, and there is a suggestion of a filling defect at this site. An air-contrast study is ordered for the following day. However, the patient refuses to undergo any further study, as he is very sore and does not want anything further done.

STUDY QUESTIONS

3 Would you be satisfied that a potential serious diagnosis has been ruled out? How would you deal with the patient's noncompliance, and what would you say to the family?

4 If an air-contrast barium enema study that was technically satisfactory still showed a questionable filling defect, are there any other studies that may help you in pursuit of a diagnosis?

SUBSEQUENT COURSE

The patient is admitted to the hospital for further studies. A napkin-ring constricting adenocarcinoma of the proximal sigmoid loop is visualized, and a biopsy specimen is taken.

STUDY QUESTIONS

5 What is the rate of incidence of colon cancer? What parts of the colon are most commonly involved?

6 Discuss the epidemiology of colon neplasia, its relationship to colonic polyps, and the relative results of surgical treatment with expected outcomes.

7 Discuss the modes of spread and extension of colon cancer. Define the Dukes' and tumor-node-metastases (TNM) classifications used to describe the extent of disease.

8 Compare and contrast signs and symptoms of a cancer of the right side as opposed to the left side of the colon.

9 What are the operations most often performed for cancers (1) of the right colon, (2) of the left colon, and (3) of the rectum? What is the significance of (1) perforation and (2) obstruction in the decision as to choice of operation?

10 What does it mean when one describes "staged procedure" for colon cancer? How does one differentiate between acute diverticulitis with perforation and a perforated colon cancer?

11 After colon resection for cancer, what factors determine who is a candidate for "adjuvant therapy"? What are the roles of cryosurgery, chemotherapy, and radiation therapy in cancer of the colon and rectum?

12 Describe how one would follow up a patient with colon resection for cancer. What laboratory and x-ray studies are appropriate and at what intervals?

Rectal Pain

A 28-year-old man presents to the emergency department with 36 hours of severe throbbing in his rectum. He denies any rectal bleeding and history of previous difficulties in the area.

STUDY QUESTIONS

1 What very specific questions might you ask, the answers to which may assist in making a diagnosis?

2 List the differential diagnosis of this patient's presenting symptoms.

3 Describe the physical findings for each of your listed diagnoses.

4 Perianal disease may be related to other illnesses. Name and describe them.

5 What is the management of pruritus ani?

6 What are initial and follow-up management of fissures, fistulae, and hemorrhoids?

7 When is surgical intervention appropriate, and what operative procedure is done in each of these entities? Are ambulatory options available?

8 How are the special problems of postoperative anorectal surgery managed?

Melena

A 68-year-old man was transferred from the State Psychiatric Hospital to the medical service with a history of passing black, tarry stools for 1 week prior to transfer. Due to Alzheimer's disease (chronic cerebral atrophy) the patient did not talk and there was no other history available on transfer. While in the medical service, the patient required five blood transfusions to raise his hematocrit from 23 to 28%. His vital signs remained stable and abdominal findings revealed no tenderness or rebound. He had good peristaltic sounds. Systemic examination was within normal limits. While on the ward, he continued to drop his hematocrit and pass black bowel movements.

STUDY QUESTIONS

1 Which of the following do you perform to come to a diagnosis?:
  (*a*) Pass a nasogastric (NG) tube and check the NG aspirate;
  (*b*) Schedule an upper GI series;
  (*c*) Do a barium enema.

2 The patient continues to have guaiac-positive, black, tarry stools. Which of the following lists shows the correct priority for ordering tests?:
  (*a*) Red cell scan, arteriography, barium enema, upper GI series, colonoscopy;
  (*b*) Colonoscopy, arteriography, barium enema, upper GI series;
  (*c*) Barium enema, colonoscopy, arteriography, upper GI series.

The colonoscopy was not adequate, as the bowel was not well prepared. However, a few openings of diverticula were seen. The arteriogram did not show any angiodysplastic disorders or bleeding points. The barium enema showed diverticulosis. As the patient continued to require transfusions to maintain his hematocrit above 30%, it was decided to explore him.

STUDY QUESTIONS

3 On exploration you would proceed to perform which of the following?:
   (*a*) A total proctocolectomy;
   (*b*) A segmental colectomy, removing all sites of diverticulae;
   (*c*) Blind colotomies to determine the site of bleeding;
   (*d*) A sub-total colectomy.

SUBSEQUENT COURSE

Postoperatively, the patient did well and had no complications and was transferred to the State Hospital.

STUDY QUESTIONS

4 What do you think are the most common causes of bleeding from the lower GI tract?:
   (*a*) Diverticulosis;
   (*b*) Angioplastic malformation;
   (*c*) Bleeding duodenal ulcer;
   (*d*) Colonic cancers.

Tender Left Lower Quadrant Mass

An 82-year-old, active, independent retired banker collapses in his apartment and is discovered in an incoherent state by his daughter the next day. He is brought to the emergency room, where he is noted to be pale, diaphoretic, mildly disoriented, and with BP 80/40 mm Hg, P 102 and irregular, R 22, and T 39.5°C (103°F). Crystalloid infusions are begun.

Examination of the abdomen reveals a tender mass in the left lower quadrant. Chest and abdominal x-rays and ECG are all negative except for atrial fibrillation by ECG.

STUDY QUESTIONS

1 Give a *concise* differential diagnosis of "collapse" in the elderly.

2 How would the diagnosis of septic shock be made?

3 What are your working diagnosis and your initial diagnostic and therapeutic plans? Give detailed admission orders (intensive care unit vs. ward, invasive monitoring, tests, drugs, intravenous fluids).

4 What are the three most common intraabdominal causes of occult sepsis in the elderly?

5 This patient promptly responds to your initial management of his septic shock, is now hemodynamically stable, and is ready for a diagnostic workup to demonstrate the cause of the sepsis. What tests would you do and when?

Tender Left Lower Quadrant Mass (Continued)

The patient in case 13-4 improves in the intensive care unit and on intravenous fluids, broad-spectrum antibiotics, and assiduous critical care. On his 5th hospital day he undergoes a limited, low-pressure barium enema without a bowel preparation, which reveals typical evidence of acute and chronic sigmoid diverticulitis with possible intramesenteric perforation and abscess.

STUDY QUESTIONS

1 What is the typical natural history of sigmoid diverticulitis in elderly adults? What treatment, if any, is usually necessary?

2 Define diverticulosis, diverticulitis, acute diverticulitis, and recurrent versus chronic diverticulitis.

3 What is the treatment for each of the above? When is surgery indicated?

4 Does this patient require an operation? If so, what surgical options are available for a patient with perforated diverticulitis with abscess ("intramural" abscess)?

5 What are the most common complications of this disease and of its surgical treatment?

6 Define one-, two-, and three-stage resections for diverticulitis. How did the historical evolution of these procedures reflect the pathophysiology of the disease? What is the Hartmann procedure?

7 What are the specific indications, techniques, morbidity, mortality, and end results in staged resections for diverticulitis?

8 What is the proper operation for this patient? Postoperative plans? Long-term plans?

9 Explain the above in clear, concise layman's terms, avoiding medical jargon as you would to the patient at a family conference when you explain the diagnosis and the need for operation. Include a sketch of the planned operation.

Colonic Obstruction

An 83-year-old female patient on the medical service develops gradual abdominal distention 6 days after placement of her transvenous pacemaker for sick sinus syndrome. When you see her she is markedly distended, tympanitic, tender, with leukocytosis, and evidence on x-ray of a closed-loop obstruction including a cutoff of gas at the sigmoid level. A nasogastric tube is passed and appropriate fluids are administered, but after 4 hours of observation she is worse. Surgical intervention is necessary, but because the patient is frail, inadequately prepared, and not throughly evaluated, a loop transverse colostomy is performed with local anesthesia.

STUDY QUESTIONS

1 What is a stoma?

2 Compare and contrast each of the following with respect to their indications and how effectively each accomplishes *decompression* and *diversion* of the fecal stream:
   (*a*) Tube cecostomy;
   (*b*) Transverse-loop colostomy;
   (*c*) "Double barrel" transverse colostomy;
   (*d*) End sigmoid colostomy;
   (*e*) Mucous fistula;
   (*f*) Ileostomy.

3 When the patient recovers from her colostomy operation and from her colonic obstruction, what, if anything, should follow?

4 Is this patient's colostomy temporary or permanent? Does she irrigate it? How is the appliance (bag) attached? What instructions do you give the patient about aftercare and follow-up?

Anemia and an Abdominal Mass

A 65-year-old woman is brought to the emergency room because of progressive weakness and an episode of near syncope 1 hour ago. Physical examination reveals a pale, moderately ill-appearing elderly woman in no acute distress with BP 120/70 mm Hg, P 90 and regular, and R 14. Abdominal examination shows a vague mass in the right lower quadrant (RLQ), and the stool is guaiac 2+. For the past 6 months she has been on pills for anemia prescribed for her personal physician. Her hematocrit is 20%.

STUDY QUESTIONS

1 Describe the appropriate workup for anemia in a post-menopausal woman.

2 How would you proceed with the evaluation of the RLQ mass and positive stool quaiac?

3 What do you expect to find?

4 What is the appropriate treatment?

<h1>SECTION 14</h1>

Biliary Tract

Michael D. Wertheimer, M.D.

REFERENCES

1. *Essentials of General Surgery*—Lawrence: Chapter 19.

2. *Principles of Surgery*—Schwartz: Chapter 31.

3. *Textbook of Surgery*—Sabiston: Chapter 38.

4. *Clinical Surgery*—Davis: Chapters 25 and 49.

5. *Current Surgical Diagnosis and Treatment*—Way: Chapter 27.

6. *Essentials of Surgery*—Sabiston: Chapter 28.

7. *Principles of Basic Surgical Practice*—James et al.: Chapter 20.

Acute Right Upper Quadrant Abdominal Pain with Fever and Vomiting

A 63-year-old man with a past medical history of angina pectoris presents to the emergency room with severe upper abdominal pain radiating to the right scapula. The pain has been continuous for approximately 3 hours and has been associated with one episode of bilious vomiting.

On physical examination, the patient is diaphoretic, sitting in bed, and has right upper quadrant tenderness without rebound. His temperature is 38.4°C (101.1°F) orally, and his pulse is 100.

STUDY QUESTIONS

1 What is the differential diagnosis for this man's abdominal pain?

2 What additional points in the history, physical examination, and simple laboratory tests availabe in the emergency room would allow you to arrive at a working diagnosis?

3 What is your therapeutic plan for this patient for the first 4 hours? For the next 12 hours? For the subsequent 24 hours?

4 Discuss the various diagnostic modalities appropriate to this situation. Prepare an algorithm (decision tree) for the diagnosis and management of this patient from admission to definitive treatment.

Acute Right Upper Quadrant Abdominal Pain Without Fever or Vomiting

A 37-year-old obese woman presents to the emergency room with her first episode ever of severe right-side upper abdominal pain without fever, nausea, vomiting, or other GI dysfunction. Her past medical history is entirely normal. While she is waiting to be seen, the pain gradually subsides. The physical examination reveals only minimal residual right upper quadrant tenderness.

STUDY QUESTIONS

1 What is the likely diagnosis for this patient?

2 What further workup and disposition are indicated?

3 How would your workup and disposition be altered if the patient had fever, leukocytosis, and marked right upper quadrant guarding?

4 What is the pathophysiology of acute cholecystitis, and how does it differ clinically from acute biliary colic?

5 What are your advice and management plans for the patient with acute biliary colic, and the one with acute cholecystitis?

Asymptomatic Gallstones

A 67-year-old healthy man comes to you complaining of heartburn for 1 week. The upper GI series you ordered shows no abnormalities in the esophagus, stomach, or duodenum. Five 1-cm radiopaque gallstones were seen. The patient has come to your office for the report and your advice.

STUDY QUESTIONS

1 What are asymptomatic gallstones? How does one ever know that stones and pain syndromes are related cause and effect?

2 Would an ultrasound, an HIDA scan, or an oral cholecystogram distinguish between stones found in a normal versus a diseased gallbladder? How does each of these tests portray the gallbladder, and what are the indications and limitations of each?

3 What is the natural history of asymptomatic gallstones?

4 What are the epidemiology and etiology of gallstones?

5 What are the complications of neglected gallstone disease?

6 Using risk-benefit analysis, devise a treatment plan to advise this highly intelligent but skeptical patient.

Jaundice

A 75-year-old man who had undergone an uncomplicated cholecystectomy and common duct exploration 15 years prior to this admission now presents with deep jaundice, weight loss, and anorexia.

STUDY QUESTIONS

1 What are your admission orders? (vital signs, diet, intravenous fluids, antibiotics, laboratory tests).

2 What is the differential diagnosis and laboratory workup of the jaundiced patient? What results would you expect? Differentiate extrahepatic from intrahepatic biliary obstruction by using laboratory investigations.

3 Define: (*a*). Murphy's sign; (*b*). Courvoisier's sign; (*c*). Ascending cholangitis, triad of symptoms.

4 What sequence of radiographic investigations would most expeditiously and economically yield the anatomic diagnosis?

5 What are the advantages and disadvantages of endoscopic retrograde cholangiopancreatography (ERCP) versus transhepatic cholangiography (THC) in distinguishing between stone, stricture, and tumor?

6 What is the most common cause of biliary stricture? Can biliary strictures be prevented? What is the surgical treatment of biliary strictures?

7 A cholangiocarcinoma in what part of the biliary tree has the best prognosis? The worst? What is the ideal preoperative workup for such a patient? What is the best surgical treatment for cure and for palliation? What treatment results can be expected?

Pancreas

Michael D. Wertheimer, M.D.

REFERENCES

1. *Essentials of General Surgery*—Lawrence: Chapter 6.

2. *Principles of Surgery*—Schwartz: Chapter 32.

3. *Textbook of Surgery*—Sabiston: Chapter 36.

4. *Clinical Surgery*—Davis: Chapter 50.

5. *Current Surgical Diagnosis and Treatment*—Way: Chapter 28.

6. *Essentials of Surgery*—Sabiston: Chapter 29.

7. *Principles of Basic Surgical Practice*—James et al.: Chapter 40.

Massive Upper GI Bleeding

Your patient is a 38-year-old man with a vague ulcer-like history who is admitted with massive upper GI bleeding. Endoscopy shows multiple gastric and duodenal ulcers. Persistant bleeding despite maximum conservative therapy precludes further evaluation, and the patient is taken to the operating room for an emergency operation. At the time of operation multiple ulcers are noted, and a tumor mass is noted in the proximal tail of the pancreas.

STUDY QUESTIONS

1 What is the most likely diagnosis?

2 How would you confirm this?

3 What diagnostic procedures would have confirmed the diagnosis preoperatively?

4 What are your therapeutic options in this patient at this time? Which would you recommend?

5 What other syndromes are associated with pancreatic tumors? Describe the pathogenesis and management of each.

Progressive Jaundice with an Abdominal Mass

The 64-year-old president of your local bank comes to see you with a 2-month history of mild abdominal discomfort, weight loss, and a yellow discoloration of his eyes noted by his wife yesterday. He has recently noted that his urine has become dark and his stools have become light.

On physical examination he is obviously jaundiced. His abdomen is soft and nontender, with a mass in the right upper quadrant that moves with respiration. Rectal examination is negative with guaiac-negative, clay-colored stool in the ampulla.

Laboratory studies are normal except for liver function tests that show a total bilirubin of 5.6 mg/dl with 3.6 mg/dl direct reacting, an alkaline phosphatase of 386 units (N: 30–115) with normal amylase, albumin, and prothrombin time.

STUDY QUESTIONS

1 What are your preliminary diagnosis and differential diagnosis?

2 How would you proceed to establish the diagnosis definitively?

3 What do you think the right upper quadrant mass represents?

4 Outline your plan of treatment for each of the three major possible diagnoses.

5 Describe the operations involved in each.

6 What is the prognosis of each condition?

7 How would you differentiate between obstructive, hemolytic, and hepatocellular forms of jaundice?

Chronic Recurrent Pancreatitis

A 44-year-old man with documented recurrent attacks of pancreatitis comes to you for renewal of his pain medication prescription for chronic abdominal pain. Despite his symptoms, he has continued to drink and has also become dependent on pain medication.

On examination he is a thin, unkempt man complaining of abdominal pain. He does have some abdominal tenderness, but his serum amylase is normal. He states that he has lost about 25 lb over the past year, and confirms that he is eating less and drinking more because of the pain. His stools are foul smelling and float in the toilet bowl. An abdominal X-ray examination shows marked pancreatic calcification.

STUDY QUESTIONS

1 What is the presumed diagnosis?

2 Explain the pathophysiology of his symptoms.

3 What nonoperative forms of treatment are available? Operative?

4 If operation is selected, what procedures are available? Describe them. Is any further preoperative workup necessary?

5 What is the success rate of each of the above procedures? What are the complications of these operations?

Severe Abdominal Pain

A 28-year-old auto mechanic shows up in your emergency room at 4:00 AM with severe abdominal pain. He is a binge drinker and was at a party the night before when he consumed a large amount of beer. He vomited twice before coming to the hospital.

On admission he was in severe pain with marked abdominal tenderness and spasm in the upper abdomen. Vital signs were stable except for a tachycardia. Serum amylase was 3400 IU, bilirubin 1.5 mg/dl, NA^+ 140 mEq/liter, K^+ 4.2 mEq/liter, Cl^- 95 mEq/liter, CO_2^- mEq/liter, and Ca^{++} 7.2 mEq/liter. Kidney, ureter, bladder (KUB) and upright abdomen x-rays showed a dilated loop of small bowel in the left upper quadrant.

STUDY QUESTIONS

1 What is your initial diagnosis?

2 How would you initially manage this patient?

3 What are the complications associated with the acute phase of this disease? How are they managed?

SUBSEQUENT COURSE

Initially your patient responded to your conservative treatment with a decrease in his abdominal pain, return of bowel sounds, and return of laboratory studies toward normal. Oral feedings were resumed on the 10th hospital day, but his pain returns and his amylase again begins to rise. A fullness is noted in his epigastrium. After another week, an epigastric mass is definitely present that appears cystic on abdominal ultrasound and measures $10 \times 6 \times 6$ cm.

STUDY QUESTIONS

4 What do you think has happened?

5 What are other causes of recurrent hyperamylasemia?

6 What is your current plan of treatment considering this new development?

7 What is the role of operative treatment in the management of this complication?

8 When would you recommend operation? What kind of an operation?

Breast and Adrenals

Michael D. Wertheimer, M.D.

REFERENCES

1. *Essentials of General Surgery*—Lawrence: Chapter 21.

2. *Principles of Surgery*—Schwartz: Chapters 15 and 37.

3. *Textbook of Surgery*—Sabiston: Chapters 22 and 26.

4. *Clinical Surgery*—Davis: Chapters 42 and 66.

5. *Current Surgical Diagnosis and Treatment*—Way: Chapters 18 and 35.

6. *Essentials of Surgery*—Sabiston: Chapters 17 and 20.

7. *Principles of Basic Surgical Practice*—James et al.: Chapters 14 and 27.

Nipple Discharge and a Nodular Breast

A 53-year-old Hispanic woman with a negative past medical history and negative family history complains of painful nodularity and serious discharge from the left breast.

STUDY QUESTION

1 Since pain, lumps, and nipple discharge are common symptoms of breast disease, and since approximately 10 to 11% of women in the United States develop breast cancer, what features of the history and physical examination would you specifically seek and record to differentiate the patient with serious pathology from the one with an innocuous physiologic aberration?

Post-Breast-Biopsy Management

At the time of the first postoperative office visit after her recent ambulatory breast biopsy, your patient wishes to understand what the significance of the pathology is, what the prognosis is, what (if any) further treatment is necessary, and how to prevent or influence a similar recurrence.

STUDY QUESTIONS

For each of the following five patients whose final pathology reports are listed, answer the questions posed above by role-playing in an office setting, avoiding medical jargon as much as possible.

1 Sclerosing adenosis.

2 Atypical ductal epithelial hyperplasia.

3 Gross cystic disease.

4 Lobular carcinoma in situ (lobular neoplasia).

5 Infiltrating ductal carcinoma.

Breast Mass

A 46-year-old Caucasian woman, mother of two, actively menstruating, whose premenopausal sister has been treated for breast cancer, has never been screened for breast cancer. She now presents with a finger tip-sized, rock-hard mass in her right breast. The patient is a highly intelligent Ph.D. biochemist who comes to the first office visit in a very anxious state with her engineer husband.

STUDY QUESTIONS

1 What are the current American Cancer Society guidelines for screening of adult women in the United States for breast cancer?

2 What data show that screening for breast cancer is effective and improves survival in screened populations?

3 What is multiphasic breast cancer screening?

4 What is this woman's diagnosis and clinical stage?

5 How will you counsel her with regard to the diagnosis and what will be your next immediate steps in the office?

6 What treatment options will you offer her? What exactly will you say, how will you say it, and how will you structure the consultation between you, the patient, and the husband?

7 What short-term plan of precise steps will you lay out for the patient for the next few days?

8 When will you schedule your next office visit for the patient? What additional information will you want to have? Whom do you want to be present at the office visit with the patient?

Positive Aspiration Biopsy of Breast

A 38-year-old female pathologist, mother of two small children, has malignant cells on fine-needle aspiration biopsy of a suspicious 1.5-cm breast mass.

STUDY QUESTIONS

1 How will you tell her the news? Exactly what will you say?

2 Does she need an open surgical biopsy to corroborate the cytology before you discuss treatment with her?

3 How would you have set up this second meeting, and whom would you have planned in advance to include?

4 What metastatic workup, if any, is necessary?

5 What is the basis of local versus systemic treatment of premenopausal breast cancer?

6 What are the current standards of acceptable local treatment for this patient? How will you explain this to a highly intelligent, medically sophisticated patient?

7 Under what circumstances would she benefit from "adjuvant' systemic treatment?

8 What is the current consensus regarding the indications and efficacy of adjuvant systemic chemotherapy in premenopausal patients?

9 What is total rehabilitation of the breast cancer patient? What does it consist of?

10 Does breast reconstruction influence survival?

Miscellaneous Breast Lesions

Instructions: Discuss each study question for each of the following cases.

a. A 72-year-old woman with a 5-cm rock-hard, fixed-mass left axillary tail, no palpable axillary nodes.

b. A 51-year-old woman, asymptomatic, who has an abnormality on a screening mammogram.

c. A 46-year-old woman whose mother and sister have premenopausal breast cancer has gross fibrocystic disease of both breasts with nondiagnostic mammographic pattern; biopsy of suspicious lesions shows "benign fibrocystic disease with severe dysplasia and atypia."

d. A 32-year-old lactating woman who develops a painful breast mass.

e. A 31-year-old woman with negative past medical history and family history for breast disease who has a solitary outer quadrant lesion and recent onset of blood-tinged nipple discharge.

STUDY QUESTIONS

1 What are the essentials of the physical examination and assessment of breast lumps?

2 Make a clinical differential diagnosis of each breast lesion.

3 Discuss clinical staging in each case with respect to prognosis.

4 What is your plan of diagnosis and treatment of each patient?

5 What should the preoperative survey consist of for each patient? (Discuss techniques to determine the extent of disease and evaluation of occult systemic metastases.)

6 What are the surgical and emotional considerations in biopsy of suspicious lesions?

7 Discuss pathologic diagnosis and differential diagnosis.

8 What is minimal (stage 0) breast cancer? What is high-risk benign disease?

9 What are the modalities of treatment of potentially curable breast cancer?

10 What is estrogen and progesterone receptor status, and how might it influence prognosis and planning of adjuvant therapy? What is the National Surgical Adjuvant Breast Project (NSABP)?

11 What are the psychosocial implications of mastectomy, and what supports are available to deal with them?

12 What are the indications for breast reconstruction?

13 What is the natural history of untreated or neglected breast cancer?

14 Discuss the treatment of locally advanced, recurrent, and disseminated breast cancer (surgery, radiotherapy, endocrinotherapy, chemotherapy, immunotherapy).

15 Is screening for breast cancer effective or worthwhile? What is the relevant epidemiology?

Hypertension

A 56-year-old female banker is undergoing a workup for the recent onset of hypertension. Her astute internist believes she has a Cushingoid appearance.

STUDY QUESTIONS

1 What is Cushing's syndrome? Cushing's disease?

2 What is the normal physiology of the adrenal cortical hormones (glucocorticoids, mineralocorticolds, sex hormones)?

3 Contrast primary adrenal dysfunction (e.g., adrenal tumor) with secondary adrenal dysfunction (due to pituitary tumor and excessive adrenocorticotropic hormone) (ACTH).

4 Describe the physical findings and laboratory abnormalities in Cushing's disease.

5 How does the dexamethasone suppression test confirm this diagnosis and discriminate between Cushing's disease and syndrome?

6 What is the pathology in Cushing's syndrome, and what is the treatment?

7 What is the pathophysiology of primary hyperaldosteronism (Conn's syndrome)?

Suprarenal Mass

A 33-year-old traveling salesman, whose only significant past medical history includes mild essential hypertension, collapses with abdominal pain and hypotension while away from home. There is no history of trauma. In the emergency room he is found to have a distended abdomen, hypotension, and a positive abdominal tap. At exploration, bleeding from a large (15-cm) right retroperitoneal (suprarenal) mass is noted. Pathology of the resected specimen reveals a "ruptured malignant pheochromocytoma."

STUDY QUESTIONS

1 Describe the physiology and pathophysiology of the adrenal medulla.

2 What is the usual clinical presentation of pheochromocytoma? What are its typical symptoms?

3 What is the biochemical evaluation of suspected pheochromocytoma? How is the tumor located? What possible locations can they occur in?

4 What are the preoperative preparation and the operative technique for patients with pheochromocytoma?

5 Does this patient have benign or malignant pheochromocytoma? What are the clinical course and the prognosis of each?

Thyroid and Parathyroid

Michael D. Wertheimer, M.D.

REFERENCES

1. *Essentials of General Surgery*—Lawrence: Chapter 22.

2. *Principles of Surgery*—Schwartz: Chapter 38.

3. *Textbook of Surgery*—Sabiston: Chapters 24 and 25.

4. *Clinical Surgery*—Davis: Chapter 65.

5. *Current Surgical Diagnosis and Treatment*—Way: Chapter 17.

6. *Essentials of Surgery*—Sabiston: Chapters 18 and 19.

7. *Principles of Basic Surgical Practice*—James et al.: Chapters 28, 29, and 30.

Enlarged Thyroid Gland

A 24-year-old woman presents in the second trimester of her pregnancy with anxiety, tachycardia, and hypertension. She complains of feeling hot all the time, and her hair is thinning.

Examination reveals a thin woman with exophthalmos bilaterally and lid lag. Her neck examination demonstrates a diffuse goiter.

STUDY QUESTIONS

1 You make the presumptive diagnosis of thyrotoxicosis. What is your management plan? What are the indications for surgery in hyperthyroidism?

SUBSEQUENT COURSE

You take this patient to the operating room after "appropriate" preparation for thyroid surgery. She has a hypertensive crisis and develops congestive heart failure in the recovery room.

STUDY QUESTIONS

2 How do you treat thyroid storm? What are the complications that you most anticipate?

3 The patient is extubated on the 9th postoperative day and complains of hoarseness. What are some of the possible causes? How would you confirm your diagnosis? What would the prognosis be for recovery?

A Lump in the Thyroid

A 20-year-old man presents with a solitary thyroid nodule. Thyroid scan shows it to be "cold."

STUDY QUESTIONS

1 List the indications for exploration of a solitary thyroid nodule.

2 Thyroid lobectomy reveals amyloid in the specimen, and pathology confirms the diagnosis of medullary cancer of the thyroid. What procedure should be completed?

3 Postoperatively the patient develops tingling in his fingers and carpopedal spasm. What are your diagnosis and plan?

4 In patients with medullary cancer of the thyroid, one is concerned that the patient may have hereditary multiple endocrine adenomatosis (MEA) syndrome. What do MEA-1 and MEA-2 comprise?

Hypercalcemia

A 40-year-old woman is referred to your office with hypercalcemia.

STUDY QUESTIONS

1 What is the differential diagnosis of hypercalcemia?

2 What are the indications for operation in hypercalcemia?

3 Patients with hypercalcemia secondary to primary hyperparathyroidism may have a chloride : phosphorus ratio of over 33 : 1 and a mild hyperchloremia metabolic acidosis. Explain.

A Mass in the Neck

A 42-year-old white male patient presents to your office with the complaint of a nodule in the right neck for 4 weeks with increasing size and mild tenderness. He admits smoking two packs of cigarettes per day for 25 years and regularly ingesting alcohol in moderate quantities (6 beers and 2 to 4 shots of whiskey per day). The patient admits slight discomfort in the right ear on swallowing, but denies sore throat, dysphagia, and odynophagia.

Physical examination reveals a right midjugular chain node approximately 2 to 2 1/2 cm in diameter and mildly to moderately tender but mobile.

STUDY QUESTIONS

1 Describe the workup of such a neck mass. Start with the history and physical findings, proceed to diagnostic and laboratory tests, and conclude with the radiologic and operative treatment.

2 Estimate the cost of each step of this evaluation.

3 If all the above tests are negative and open biopsy of the node reveals a malignancy, described how you would proceed in each of the four cell types listed below: (*a*). Squamous carcinoma; (*b*). Anaplasatic carcinoma; (*c*). Lymphoma; (*d*). Melanoma.

4 What is the most likely site of a primary tumor with a neck node presenting above the supraclavicular area?

5 What percentage of primary tumors have a neck node as an initial symptoms (i.e., tonsil, thyroid, etc.).

6 Describe the lymphatic drainage of the head and neck and the most likely primary site of malignancy or inflammation relative to the presenting neck nodes for each of the major and minor triangles of the neck.

7 List the most common benign tumors in adults. In children.

8 List neck masses of: (*a*). Traumatic origin; (*b*). Congenital origin; (*c*). Inflammatory or infectious origin.

9 List the most common thyroid malignancies and describe the workup of a nodule that is felt to be contained within the thyroid tissue.

10 List the variance modalities of treatment indicated for the various thyroid tumors.

Asymptomatic Solitary Thyroid Nodule

A 42-year-old female journalist is found to have a 1.5-cm asymptomatic nodule in the right lobe of her thyroid gland on her yearly health maintenance examination. She is clinically euthyroid.

STUDY QUESTIONS

1 What are the salient findings that must be sought during the physical examination of such a lesion? How is a proper thyroid examination performed?

2 What laboratory examinations—including what specific thyroid function tests—are indicated, and what results do you anticipate?

3 What is the differential diagnosis of an asymptomatic "cold" nodule in a young woman?

4 Compare and contrast the indications for, risks, success rate, and cost of outpatient fine-needle aspiration cytology, out-patient "Trucut" core-needle biopsy, and inpatient open surgical biopsy.

5 Assuming the diagnosis based on fine-needle biopsy of the statistically most-likely pathology, what is the correct treatment?

6 What are the natural history, treatment, and expected prognosis of all of the lesions in your differential diagnosis?

7 What long-term follow-up and endocrine therapy might be necessary for this lesion?

Liver

John B. Herrmann, M.D.

REFERENCES

1. *Essentials of General Surgery*—Lawrence: Chapter 23.

2. *Principles of Surgery*—Schwartz: Chapter 30.

3. *Textbook of Surgery*—Sabiston: Chapter Chapter 34.

4. *Clinical Surgery*—Davis: Chapter 48.

5. *Current Surgical Diagnosis and Treatment*—Way: Chapter 25.

6. *Essentials of Surgery*—Sabiston: Chapter 34.

7. *Principles of Basic Surgical Practice*—James et al.: Chapters 20 and 21.

Tender Liver Mass

A 14-year-old boy underwent an appendectomy 10 days ago for a ruptured appendicitis with abscess formation. Despite antibiotic therapy, he has remained febrile and ill with an elevated blood count. This morning he complained of upper abdominal pain, and you noted a tender, vague upper abdominal mass with scleral icterus. A CT scan fails to reveal any evidence of an intraperitoneal abscess, but does show a mass in the right lobe of the liver.

STUDY QUESTIONS

1 What is the likely diagnosis?

2 Discuss the pathogenesis of this lesion.

3 How would you confirm your suspected diagnosis?

4 How would you treat this lesion? Are there any alternatives?

5 How could this problem have been prevented?

6 Are there other causes of this type of lesion? Discuss differences in treatment (if any).

Massive Upper GI Bleeding

A 48-year-old known alcoholic presents at your emergency room having vomited a copious amount of blood. He is hypotensive and clinically jaundiced with hepatosplenomegaly and spider angiomata. Rectal examination is negative with tarry, guaiac 4+ stool in the ampulla.

STUDY QUESTIONS

1 What immediate therapeutic measures would you recommend?

2 What is the most likely cause of bleeding in this patient? What are the other possibilities? How would you determine the specific site and cause of bleeding? Is this important?

3 What is Child's classification? How does it influence therapy?

4 Assuming the diagnosis of portal hypertension and bleeding esophageal varices secondary to nutritional cirrhosis of the liver and moderately well-preserved liver function, what immediate and definite courses of treatment would you recommend? What are the various alternatives?

5 Describe the various types of operations that have been commonly used in this situation. What are the advantages and disadvantages of each?

6 Would a platelet count of 54,000/ml influence your treatment? The presence of ascites? Severe encephalopathy?

7 What is the overall prognosis?

Intractable Ascites

A 56-year-old patient of yours with cirrhosis has gradually developed massive ascites despite medical treatment with a low-salt diet and diuretics. He is admitted to the hospital for futher evaluation and treatment.

Physical examination reveals tense ascites, a protuberant umbilical hernia filled with fluid, moderate muscle wasting, and minimal jaundice. Laboratory studies show a bilirubin of 2.6 mg/dl, albumin of 2.2 gm/dl, blood urea nitrogen (BUN) of 80 mg/dl, creatinine of 4.2 mg/dl, and normal coagulation studies.

After 2 weeks of intensive in-hospital therapy, his weight and ascites are unchanged and his creatinine is now 5.6 mg/dl.

STUDY QUESTIONS

1 Describe the pathophysiology of ascites in advanced liver disease.

2 What is the hepatorenal syndrome? Does this patient have it?

3 In view of the failure of medical therapy, is there any surgical procedure available?

4 What are the complications of operative treatment? How would you best avoid or treat them?

5 What is the overall prognosis of patients with this condition with or without surgery?

6 What is the significance of the umbilical hernia?

7 If this patient should die, could he be considered as a kidney donor for transplantation? Why?

Hepatomegaly

The patient is a 47-year-old former alcoholic who was diagnosed as having cirrhosis of the liver 10 years ago, and since then has completely abstained from alcohol. Since then he has done well until about 3 months ago, when he began to feel weak and tired and was recently noted to be jaundiced. His primary physician noted a newly enlarged liver, and a liver-spleen scan showed a mass in the right lobe of the liver. He is referred to you for advice and treatment.

STUDY QUESTIONS

1 What is your differential diagnosis?

2 What further studies would you suggest to determine the etiology of this lesion?

3 What form of treatment would you suggest?

4 List the major primary and secondary tumors of the liver and their treatment.

5 Describe the segmental anatomy of the liver and its importance in liver resection.

6 What are the major complications of liver resection, and how can they be treated?

Spleen

John B. Herrmann, M.D.

REFERENCES

1. *Essentials of General Surgery*—Lawrence: Chapter 4.

2. *Principles of Surgery*—Schwartz: Chapter 33.

3. *Textbook of Surgery*—Sabiston: Chapter 37.

4. *Clinical Surgery*—Davis: Chapter 63.

5. *Current Surgical Diagnosis and Treatment*—Way: Chapter 29.

6. *Essentials of Surgery*—Sabiston: Chapter 30.

7. *Principles of Basic Surgical Practice*—James et al.: Chapter 19.

Abdominal and Chest Trauma

A 42-year-old male musician driving home from a late performance skids on ice and crashes, his car spinning into a utility pole. The "cave in" injury to the left side of the car pins the victim in the vehicle and requires extrication by emergency medical technicians, which takes 40 minutes. The patient is transiently dazed but awake, alert, and oriented during transport and arrives in the emergency room with BP 80/60 mm Hg, P 120, and R 23, and complaining of chest and abdominal pain.

STUDY QUESTIONS

1 Discuss initial resuscitation and the primary survey of this multiply injured patient.

2 There is prompt restoration of blood pressure with crystalloid infusion. The chest x-ray is normal except for fractures of ribs 9 and 10 posteriorly. There is microscopic hematuria. What is your decision tree now?

3 What are the five most common injuries—in order of frequency—to left upper quadrant structures? What are three mechanisms of injury?

4 Draw an algorithm for a reasonable and rapid clinical, laboratory, and radiologic assessment of this patient's injury.

HOSPITAL PROGRESS

The patient continues hemodynamically stable and is found to have no other injuries except the left 9th and 10th rib fractures outside of the abdomen. A CT scan of the abdomen reveals a shattered spleen (type IV), a contused left kidney, swelling in the tail of the pancreas, and free blood in the pelvis.

5 Is there a role for ''conservative'' (nonoperative) management of such a patient? What are the currently accepted standards for splenic preservation?

6 What is the operative strategy in patients with blunt trauma to the left upper abdominal quadrant? Discovery and repair of associated injuries?

7 What are the potential hematologic and immunologic consequences of splenectomy? Surveillance? Prophylaxis?

Left Upper Quadrant Fullness

A 23-year-old female graduate student notes the gradual onset of fatigue, unusually heavy menstrual periods, easy bruisability, and upper abdominal pain. Initial evaluation at the student health service reveals scattered ecchymoses, some petechiae, left upper quadrant fullness, Hct 29%, platelet count 35,000, and serum bilirubin mg/dl.

STUDY QUESTIONS

1 What is your initial differential diagnosis?

2 What additional points in the history are important and what *important* physical findings (positive and negative) are relevant?

3 What is the pathophysiology and immunopathology of adult hypersplenism? What cardinal features of the peripheral blood smear might differentiate a secondary (e.g., drug-induced) thrombocytopenia from idiopathic thrombocytopenia purpura (ITP) or acute leukemia?

4 What is the proper medical management of idiopathic thrombocytopenia purpura (ITP)?

5 When is splenectomy considered appropriate in ITP?

6 What are five hematologic diagnoses sometimes considered for splenectomy?

7 What complications after splenectomy are watched for? What changes in the blood smear typically occur after splenectomy?

Vascular System

John B. Herrmann, M.D.

REFERENCES

1. *Essentials of General Surgery*—Lawrence: Chapter 25.

2. *Principles of Surgery*—Schwartz: Chapters 21, 22, and 23.

3. *Textbook of Surgery*—Sabiston: Chapters 49, 50, 51, and 53.

4. *Clinical Surgery*—Davis: Chapters 56 and 57.

5. *Current Surgical Diagnosis and Treatment*—Way: Chapters 36 and 83.

6. *Essentials of Surgery*—Sabiston: Chapters 41, 42, 43, and 31.

7 *Principles of Basic Surgical Practice*—James et al.: Chapters 33–38.

Pulsatile Epigastric Mass

A 55-year-old man with a 4-year history of mild high blood pressure is referred to your office because his family doctor felt a pulsatile mass in his abdomen.

STUDY QUESTIONS

1 What is the differential diagnosis?

2 Discuss various noninvasive methods of confirming the diagnosis of abdominal aortic aneurysm.

3 What is the natural history of an abdominal aortic aneurysm?

4 Should this patient have an aortogram?

5 If the aneurysm proves to be 6 cm in diameter, what is the appropriate management?

6 Under what circumstances might you decide not to operate electively on an abdominal aortic aneurysm?

7 Discuss the management of this patient if he presented in the emergency room with hypotension; abdominal and back pain; and a tender, diffuse, pulsatile epigastric mass.

8 Compare the operative mortality of elective aneurysm surgery with that for a ruptured aneurysm.

9 What are the major factors contributing to mortality following aneurysm surgery?

Hematochezia Following Aneurysm Surgery

A 65-year-old man comes to the emergency ward with symptoms of weakness, sweating, and passage of dark blood by bowel movements. There is a history of a previous operation for abdominal aortic aneurysm 6 years ago.

Vital signs are: BP 110/70 mm Hg, P 110 and regular, and R 18. Abdominal examination reveals a well-healed midline incision with minimal epigastric tenderness and hyperactive bowel sounds. Rectal examination shows gross dark blood. Peripheral pulses are normal. Hematocrit is 36%, WBC 10,500, normal differential.

STUDY QUESTIONS

1 What further studies would you recommend to determine the source of bleeding?

2 What are the most likely causes?

3 How would you manage each of the most likely diagnoses?

4 Could any of these conditions have been prevented? How?

Calf Pain and Tenderness

A 45-year-old laborer comes to see you because of pain in his right calf. There is no history of trauma. On physical examination he has a very prominent popliteal pulse about 3 cm in diameter and good pedal pulses. There is mild calf tenderness with no evidence of swelling.

STUDY QUESTIONS

1 What are the possible causes of the patient's symptoms of calf pain?

2 What diagnostic studies would you want to perform to confirm your diagnostic impression?

3 What treatment would you recommend?

4 What percentrage of these patients will also have other evidence of aneurysmal disease?

Intermittent Claudication

A 52-year-old mailman comes to see you because of pain and weakness in his right leg after walking about 200 ft. He has had these symptoms for about 1 year, and they have been getting worse to the point where he is having difficulty working. The pain goes away after he rests for a few minutes, and he has had no symptoms at night.

Past history reveals a myocardial infarct four year ago, stable angina pectoris, and a 50 pack/year history of smoking. The patient's father and one sister are diabetics, and his mother died of a stroke.

Physical examination shows a moderately obese middle-aged man in no distress. BP 170/100 mm Hg, P 90, R 16. A left carotid bruit, an abdominal bruit, and bilateral femoral bruits are noted. Pulses are present but diminished in the left leg. The right femoral pulse is diminished, and no distal pulses are palpable on the right.

Laboratory studies show a hematocrit of 51%, a blood sugar (random) of 184 mg/dl and a blood urea nitrogen (BUN) of 20 mg/dl. Chest x-ray is normal, and an ECG shows an old inferior myocardial infarct.

STUDY QUESTIONS

1 What are your preliminary diagnoses?

2 What further diagnostic studies are indicated?

3 What are the therapeutic alternatives available for the management of this patient?

4 What would you recommend?

5 What are the possible complications of surgical treatment, and how can they best be avoided?

6 Would your recommendations be any different if this patient was found to have the following: (*a*). An 85% stenosis of his left internal carotid artery?; (*b*). A 70% stenosis of his left anterior descending coronary artery and a complete occlusion of his right coronary artery?; (*c*). A 60% stenosis of his right renal artery?; (*d*). A 90% stenosis of his superior mesenteric artery?

7 Would your plan of diagnosis and treatment be altered if the patient had severe rest pain in his right foot with pregangrenous changes in his 4th toe? If so, how?

Acute Extremity Ischemia

A 56-year-old man is brought to the emergency ward complaining of pain, numbness, coldness, and weakness of his right leg of sudden onset 1/2 hour ago.

Initial examination reveals that the right foot is pale and cool to touch and that no arterial pulses are palpable below the groin in that leg.

STUDY QUESTIONS

1 What has happened?

2 What are the diagnostic possibilities?

3 How do your estimate the degree of ischemia and decide about the likelihood of limb loss with or without vascular reconstruction?

4 How would you establish the diagnosis?

5 What initial treatment would you institute?

6 Discuss the definitive treatment for each of the diagnostic possibilities you have listed.

Transient Aphasia and Hemiparesis

A 75-year-old man sustains a sudden episode of numbness and weakness of his right arm accompanied by difficulty speaking. By the time he sees you in the emergency room 15 minutes later, his symptomes have disappeared. On physical examination he has a left carotid bruit but no other vascular or neurologic findings.

STUDY QUESTIONS

1 What is the most likely diagnosis?

2 Describe the mechanism of transient ischemic attacks (TIAs) such as the one described above.

3 Define and differentiate TIAs, reversible ischemic neurologic disabilities (RIND), cerebrovascular accidents (CVAs), and amaurosis fugax.

4 What further diagnostic studies are indicated?

5 What is the risk of stroke in this patient?

6 What would you recommend for treatment? Are there alternatives? If so, describe them.

Postoperative Dyspnea and Cyanosis

A 59-year-old obese female patient had a total gastrectomy for carcinoma 2 days previously. She apparently was recovering well until this morning, when she suddenly became short of breath, diaphoretic, and cyanotic. When you see her she is tachypneic and complaining of pain in the left side of her chest.

STUDY QUESTIONS

1 Discuss the differential diagnosis of what happened this morning.

2 What are the risk factors in this patient for pulmonary embolus?

3 What is the most likely source for pulmonary embolism in this patient?

4 How reliable is the clinical diagnosis of deep venous thrombosis?

5 What noninvasive methods are availabe to improve the accuracy of the clinical diagnosis of deep venous thrombosis?

6 What is the best initial management of this patient?

7 What would be the indications of surgical intervention in this patient, and what type of surgery would you do?

8 What are the indications for pulmonary embolectomy? Describe the principles of the procedure.

9 Are there any types of prophylactic therapy that might have prevented this event?

Varicose Veins

A 24-year-old housewife, mother of two small children, who is now taking birth control pills, comes to your office because of bilateral varicose veins. She is bothered primarily by the appearance of the veins. She denies having previously had phlebitis.

STUDY QUESTIONS

1 What is the difference between primary and secondary varicose veins?

2 What are some of the etiologic factors favoring the development of varicose veins in this patient?

3 What treatment should this patient have?

4 Is this patient at increased risk of pulmonary embolus compared to the normal population?

5 Describe the important aspects of the surgical treatment of varicose veins.

6 What is sclerotherapy, and what is its role in the treatment of varicose veins?

Cold-Induced Hand Ischemia

A 24-year-old secretary comes to see you because of pain in her right arm associated with episodes of blanching and numbness of the fingers of her right hand associated with cold exposure. Following rewarming, her fingers become cyanotic and ruborous associated with pain.

Physical examination reveals a thin, asthenic young woman with no obvious abnormalities in her upper extremities. Peripheral pulses are all present, and no neurological signs are present.

STUDY QUESTIONS

1 What is Raynaud's phenomenon? What are some of the causes of this syndrome?

2 What additional maneuvers on physical examination might be helpful? What is Adson's test? Allen's test? Costoclavicular and hyperabduction maneuvers? Cold pressor test?

3 Describe your further diagnostic workup of this young woman.

4 Describe your management of each of the possible conditions you have listed above.

5 What is the prognosis in each case?

Blunt Vascular Trauma

An 18-year-old boy sustains a fracture dislocation of his left knee in a motorcycle accident. Upon his admission to the emergency room, his right foot is pale and pulseless.

STUDY QUESTIONS

1 What do you think has happened? Is this a common injury?

2 How would you confirm the diagnosis?

3 What is the appropriate management of this patient?

4 Describe traumatic vasospasm. How is it diagnosed and managed?

5 Are there any other blunt injuries that are likely to cause vascular impairment? How would you manage them?

Leg Swelling

A 13-year-old girl presents in your office with swelling of her right leg of 3–4 months duration. This was initially mild and subsided overnight, but lately the swelling has remained. She is otherwise a healthy, active pubescent girl.

Examination reveals 3–4 cm of swelling of her right leg and foot over the left with mild pretibial pitting. There is no calf tenderness or adenopathy.

STUDY QUESTIONS

1 List the possible causes of unilateral leg edema and indicate the most likely cause in this youngster.

2 Discuss the pathophysiology of edema and the diagnostic workup of patients with edema.

3 Discuss the treatment of lower-extremity edema in general, and the management of this particular patient.

Posttraumatic Arteriovenous Fistula

A 17-year-old boy fell while climbing a tree in his back yard, sustaining a fracture of the distal right femur. At the hospital he had good pedal pulses, and the closed reduction of the femoral fracture was successful. He recovered from the fracture and returned to playing tennis the following summer. However, when he notices that he becomes short of breath very easily, he comes to your office for help.

STUDY QUESTIONS

1 What is the differential diagnosis?

2 What physical signs might you look for if you suspected an arteriovenous fistula?

3 What is the Branham-Nicoladoni sign?

4 What would you expect this patient's resting cardiac output to be?

5 Should the patient have an arteriogram?

6 Discuss the appropriate management of this patient.

Malignant Hypertension

A 22-year-old woman presents to you with a history of severe headaches with blurring of vision. Her BP is 240/140 mm Hg and she has grade III hypertensive retinopathy. She is mildly obese and has a systolic heart murmur and an epigastric bruit.

STUDY QUESTIONS

1 List the differential diagnosis of hypertension in a young woman, giving particular attention to the surgically curable causes of hypertension.

2 What further diagnostic studies would be indicated?

3 Outline your plan of treatment for each of the possible causes of her severe hypertension.

4 What is the long-term prognosis of each of the above conditions?

Ulceration of the Ankle

A 57-year-old retired government employee developed phlebitis during an airplane trip to the Middle East in 1973. Since then he has noted varicose veins and ankle swelling. Three weeks ago he developed an ulceration on the medial aspect of his ankle.

STUDY QUESTIONS

1 What probably occurred during the airplane trip in 1983?

2 What is the difference between primary and secondary varicose veins?

3 What is the pathophysiology behind the development of the ulceration?

4 Should a venogram be part of this patient's initial management?

5 How can you tell ischemic ulcerations from those caused by venous insufficiency?

6 What is the postphlebitic syndrome?

7 Should this patient be treated with anticoagulants to protect him from pulmonary embolus?

8 What are the principles of management of venous stasis ulcers?

Transplantation

Michael D. Wertheimer, M.D.

REFERENCES

1. *Essentials of General Surgery*—Lawrence: Chapter 26.

2. *Principles of Surgery*—Schwartz: Chapter 10.

3. *Textbook of Surgery*—Sabiston: Chapter 19.

4. *Clinical Surgery*—Davis: Chapter 27.

5. *Current Surgical Diagnosis and Treatment*—Way: Chapter 49.

6. *Essentials of Surgery*—Sabiston: Chapter 15.

7. *Principles of Basic Surgery Practice*—James et al.: Chapter 12.

Brain Death

A 32-year-old laboratory technician is struck by an automobile while riding his bicycle to work. He sustains a closed head injury, and after appropriate resuscitation and thorough evaluation is stable on a respirator, yet is unresponsive in the surgical intensive care unit.

STUDY QUESTIONS

1 What are the generally accepted clinical criteria determining brain death?

2 What are the confirmatory tests used in determining brain death, and how are the possible results interpreted?

3 What would make this patient an acceptable and appropriate organ donor? How is this presented to grieving family members?

4 What laboratory studies are used to determine acceptability (compatibility) of organs for transplantation?

Organ Transplantation

A 15-year-old boy is transferred by jet, intubated and on a respirator, to a large metropolitan university organ transplant center after he has been declared legally brain dead as a result of a motor vehicle accident.

STUDY QUESTIONS

1 What immunologic matching should be done for the following organs or tissues: Kidney, liver, pancreas, heart, lung, bone, and skin?

2 Define the following:
(a) ABH blood group compatibiltity;
(b) Class I histocompatibility antigens;
(c) Class II histocompatibility antigens;
(d) Mixed lymphocyte culture (MLC) tests.

3 Describe the current methods of organ harvest and preservation for kidney, heart, liver, and cornea.

4 What are the main events and distinctions in hyperacute rejection, acute rejection, and chronic rejection?

5 What are the mechanism of action and the long-term side effects of azathioprine, prednisone, and antilymphocyte globulin, and cyclosporine when used in therapeutic doses for recipient immunosuppression?

6 What are recipient criteria for renal, cardiac, pancreatic, and hepatic transplantation?

7 What are current rates of long-term success with kidney, liver, and heart transplants?

Malignant Diseases of the Skin

John B. Herrmann, M.D.

REFERENCES

1. *Essentials of General Surgery*—Lawrence: Chapter 27.

2. *Principles of Surgery*—Schwartz: Chapters 14 and 16.

3. *Textbook of Surgery*—Sabiston: Chapters 40 and 45.

4. *Clinical Surgery*—Davis: Chapters 37, 40, and 62.

5. *Current Surgical Diagnosis and Treatment*—Way: Chapter 45.

6. *Essentials of Surgery*—Sabiston: Chapter 37.

Pigmented Lesion of the Back

A 46-year-old businessman comes to you because his wife noticed a pigmented lesion on his back while vacationing in Florida. On examination he has a 1.3-cm raised, excoriated, black pigmented lesion in his right scapular area. The lesion is freely movable, and no adenopathy or other abnormalities are noted on physical examination.

STUDY QUESTIONS

1 What is the most likely diagnosis? What is your differential diagnosis?

2 How would you confirm the diagnosis?

3 Assuming the diagnosis of melanoma, what is the significance of gross physical characteristics, histological characteristics, thickness of the lesion, and depth of invasion (Clark and Breslow's classification systems, tumor-nodes-metastasis (TNM) classification)?

4 What are your recommendations for treatment?

5 What is the prognosis?

6 What further treatment is available if primary treatment is unsuccessful and the patient returns with metastatic disease?

Discoloration of Toenail

A 26-year-old man comes to see you because of a black discoloration under his right great toenail. He initially thought this was an injury, despite being unable to recollect any trauma, but has become concerned since it has not become any better and even appears to be spreading during the past 2 months. Examination reveals a black discoloration under the medial half of the nail without swelling or tenderness. No other lesions are present, and there is no adenopathy.

STUDY QUESTIONS

1 How would you advise the patient?

2 How would you confirm the diagnosis?

3 What treatment would you recommend?

4 What would you estimate his prognosis to be?

5 One year later, after primary treatment, he returns with palpable inguinal nodes. What further treatment would you recommend, assuming workup was otherwise negative?

Groin Nodes

A 59-year-old housewife comes to see you because of a lump in her left groin. She gives a history of having multiple skin lesions removed by her dermatologist over the years by excision and electrocautery. Examination shows multiple movable nodes in the left groin and several small scars in the leg from previous excisions. Multiple nevi are present elsewhere in her body.

STUDY QUESTIONS

1 List the differential diagnoses.

2 How would you establish the correct diagnosis?

3 Are any further studies indicated?

4 Describe your recommended treatment if the histologic diagnosis turned out to be the following:
(*a*) Melanoma;
(*b*) Lymph node reactive hyperplasia;
(*c*) Squamous cell carcinoma;
(*d*) Non-Hodgkin's lymphoma, low grade;
(*e*) Hodgkin's disease, nodular sclerosing type;
(*f*) Adenocarcinoma, moderately well differentiated.

Lesion on the Nose

A 72-year-old retired businessman comes to see you because of a 7-mm nodular excoriated lesion on his nose. Biopsy confirms the diagnosis of basal cell carcinoma.

STUDY QUESTIONS

1 Describe the various methods of treatment and the advantages and disadvantages of each.

2 If surgical excision is chosen, describe the method of excision and closure of the wound.

3 What are the risks of recurrence? Of metastatic spread? Of development of similar lesions elsewhere?

4 What are the current concepts of etiology and pathogenesis? Can this kind of lesion be prevented?

Lesion on the Lip

A 56-year-old fisherman has developed a 1-cm ulcerated lesion of his lower lip. Biopsy reveals squamous cell carcinoma.

STUDY QUESTIONS

1 What are the various modalities of treatment available for this lesion?

2 Describe the surgical excision of this lesion and the method of reconstruction.

3 What is the risk of nodal metastases? Where would they likely occur? What are the treatment options available?

4 What type of follow-up would you recommend for this patient?

Malignant Diseases of Lymphatics and Soft Tissues

John B. Herrmann, M.D.

REFERENCES

1. *Essentials of General Surgery*—Lawrence: Chapter 27.

2. *Principles of Surgery*—Schwartz: Chapters 14 and 16.

3. *Textbook of Surgery*—Sabiston: Chapters 40 and 45.

4. *Clinical Surgery*—Davis: Chapters 37, 40, and 62.

5. *Current Surgical Diagnosis and Treatment*—Way: Chapter 45.

6. *Essentials of Surgery*—Sabiston: Chapter 37.

Lump in the Neck

A 19-year-old college student comes to see you because of a lump in her neck. On examination a solitary firm, movable mass is noted in the right anterior cervical region. She is otherwise asymptomatic, and the remainder of her physical examination is normal.

STUDY QUESTIONS

1 List the possible etiologies of this cervical mass. How would you work up the patient?

2 Assuming the preliminary workup is negative, describe how you would obtain a biopsy of the lesion.

3 Describe the histologic criteria for making a diagnosis of Hodgkin's disease. What are the four different categories? Describe the histologic criteria for the various types of non-Hodgkin's lymphoma.

4 If the pathologist confirms the diagnosis of Hodgkin's disease, describe the further management of the patient (staging and treatment).

5 What is the prognosis for survival for the various stages of Hodgkin's lymphoma, using current methods of treatment?

6 If the histologic diagnosis was non-Hodgkin's lymphoma, nodular type, describe the further diagnostic studies and treatment you would recommend.

Gastric Mass

A 36-year-old housewife presents with malaise, weight loss, and upper abdominal discomfort after eating. An upper GI series shows a partially obstructing mass in the antrum of the stomach. Other studies are negative. At the time of operation, a large, freely movable mass is present in the antral stomach with several large lymph nodes present in the gastrohepatic ligament. Biopsy of a node reveals a histiocytic lymphoma.

STUDY QUESTIONS

1 Should anything further be done at the time of operation? If so, what?

2 What further treatment is indicated?

3 What is the prognosis?

A Mass in the Thigh

A 34-year-old man comes to see you because of a swelling in his right thigh. He had been hit in the area playing softball 1 month previously and noticed some swelling at that time, which he assumed was due to the injury. He is now concerned that the lump is not going away but seems to be getting larger.

On examination, there is a firm, nontender, nonpulsatile 10 × 6 × 4 cm mass in the anteromedial region of the right thigh. It appears to be fixed to deeper tissues but not to the skin or bone. There are no other masses present, and no nodes are palpable. The remainder of the physical examination is normal.

STUDY QUESTIONS

1 What is your preliminary differential diagnosis? What further studies would you recommend?

2 If all other studies are not diagnostic and a biopsy appears indicated, how would you recommend that this be performed?

3 The pathologist reports a moderately differentiated soft tissue sarcoma, probably of fibrous tissue origin (fibrosarcoma). In the absence of detectable metastatic disease, describe in detail how this lesion should be treated.

4 If the diagnosis were liposarcoma, synovial cell sarcoma, angiosarcoma, or some other cell type, would the treatment or prognosis be any different?

Skin Lesions on the Leg

A 34-year-old rock musician presents in your office with multiple reddish-blue lesions of his right leg that have been progressive over the past few months. He has a history of hepatitis 2 years ago and admits to intravenous drug use.

STUDY QUESTIONS

1 What is your tentative diagnosis? How would you confirm your suspicions?

2 What is the preferred method of treating these skin lesions? What is the prognosis?

3 What other diseases may occur in association with this condition? Discuss the role of surgery in the management of these patients.

4 Are there precautions that should be taken in managing these patients?

PROBLEM INDEX